A SURGEON'S STORY

Key Insights for Today's Physician

by

Richard A. Lynn
MD, FACS, RPVI

ISBN 979-8-218-67025-2

10 9 8 7 6 5 4 3 2 1

A SURGEON'S STORY

Key Insights for Today's Physician

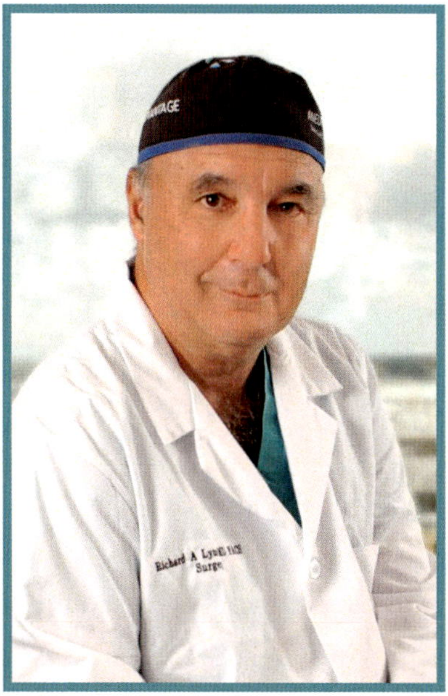

by

Richard A. Lynn

MD, FACS, RPVI

For my wife,

Margrit

whose love and endless support
helped bring this project to fruition.

For my lifelong mentor,

William Silen, MD, FACS

(1927-2022)

Emeritus Johnson & Johnson Professor of Surgery,
Harvard Medical School;
Past Chairman, Department of Surgery,
Beth Israel Hospital, Harvard Medical School
who brought out the very best in me
as a surgeon and a physician.

For my three sons,

Rabbi Shmuel (Adam) Lynn,
Rabbi Dovid (David) Lynn, and
Rabbi Dr. Yosef (Peter) Lynn

You are my whole life and my legacy.

A heartfelt thank you to the editor,
Ben Jacobson
whose dedication and meticulous attention
brought this book to life.
His unwavering commitment and
thoughtful guidance were instrumental
in seeing this project through to completion.

Reflections from a Current Medical Student

"I am inspired by your experiences, your role as a doctor, and how you conduct yourself even in the most challenging times. Words cannot express how incredible you are as a person and how much I've learned from you. I am so inspired, and my dreams of becoming a doctor have never been greater. At the end of this, I was in tears. I truly hope you know how meaningful and valued it was."

Table of Contents

Foreword

by Michael M. Meguid

꧁ Developing The Why

THERE WAS ONCE an 11-year-old boy who developed abdominal pain. His friends implored him to come out to play. Ignoring them, he fell asleep on the couch in the middle of a Sunday afternoon, curled up in a fetal position. By early evening, his mother roused him. He was cranky and complained of increasing pain. He refused food and even water. Concerned, the boy's parents called for help.

Upon arrival, the surgeon found an irritable, lethargic boy with a fever. He carefully examined the youngster. When he palpated his lower abdomen, the boy whimpered, and when he pressed more deeply on the right side and then released the pressure, the boy cried with pain.

"Your son has appendicitis and needs an emergency

operation right now," the surgeon told the concerned parents. He swooped the boy up, and, accompanied by his father, they drove to the hospital.

When the boy awoke several hours later, he was free of pain. By then, it was the middle of the night. The boy spotted something remarkable in the soft lamplight on his bedside table. He marveled at the sight of his now blackish appendix, which was floating in fluid in a small jar.

The young boy in this story was me. The event described occurred about 70 years ago, and the surgeon was my uncle. Then and there, I decided I wanted to become a surgeon so that I, too, could relieve pain and cure disease.

Interestingly, I doubt this scenario would play out the same way today. I'm almost certain of it. Many years later, I received a phone call from a very excited young man (who just happened to be my son), who was then a second-year surgical resident on his way to the Emergency Room (ER).

"Dad, I'm going to do an appendectomy," he told me.

"That's great, son," I replied, "Is it a man or a woman? How old are they?"

In response to each question, he answered that he did not know.

"Well, how do you know it's appendicitis?" I asked.

"They saw it on a CT (Computed Tomography) scan."

"You did a CT scan before examining the patient?"

"Dad! The ER resident did."

"Tell me, son," I asked him, "Did you see on the scan whether the patient's heart was on the right or left?"

"Dad, are you always going to cross-examine me when I call you about a patient?"

"Yes, son," I replied. "Nothing replaces a good history and a careful physical examination. Having a patient seek your help is a privilege, and you must provide him with the best care you can give."

Our Relationship

Such was the ethos under which Richard Lynn and I trained. In 1971, when I was a second-year resident, Dr Lynn was a diligent, curious, compassionate, and dependable surgical intern. We had both elected to rotate through the Children's Hospital in Boston, he from Beth Israel and me from what was then the Peter Bent Brigham Hospital and is now Bringham and Women's Hospital. On this rotation, we cared for critically ill children with abdominal disease, thoracic and cardiac congenital abnormalities, and those who had suffered trauma.

In this role, we assisted the "titans" of our day. This included Dr Robert E. Gross, who was the first surgeon to tie off a patent ductus arteriosus in a child's beating heart, thereby saving thousands of children who would otherwise be doomed to a limited lifespan, as well as

Dr Judah Folkman, who discovered a revolutionary new way to think about and treat cancer. Our peers were also budding giants. Among our senior residents was Dr Alberto Pena, who went on to develop the optimal procedure for the correction of anorectal malformations and cloacae in neonates, and Dr Alden Harken, a thoracic surgeon who became a Regent of the American College of Surgeons. We routinely worked 36-hour schedules, seeing patients in the ER and the clinic and operating both night and day. We depended on patient histories, physical examinations with only limited blood work, and primitive radiological examinations to guide us.

We could only dream of later developments such as CT scans, magnetic resonance imaging, and interventional radiology, and when we complained of fatigue, we were reminded that the generation of surgeons who came before us never had a night off. "You only see 50% of the cases when you work every other night" was a common refrain. They reminded us that they actually lived in the hospital, a state of affairs that led to the term "resident" physician.

Nonetheless, long live progress in the endeavor to advance the field of surgery! There will always be young people who strive to become surgeons, many because of life-changing encounters with physicians who treated their illnesses or injuries.

Richard Lynn exhibits many of the qualities that I admire in surgeons today. His many years of service and dedication to the profession, most recently as the Second Vice-President of the American College of Surgeons, render him eminently qualified to guide members of the younger generation who seek to become physicians.

Michael M. Meguid, MD, PhD, FACS, ABN, MFA
Emeritus Professor,
Surgery, Physiology/Neuroscience Program and Nutrition
State University of New York, Upstate Medical University
Surgical Metabolism and Nutrition Laboratory
Department of Surgery, University Hospital
Emeritus & Founder, Editor-In-Chief, Nutrition:
The International Journal of Applied and
Basic Nutritional Sciences
meguidm@upstate.edu

Introduction

℘ Beginnings

WHERE DOES ONE BEGIN to tell a story about a life in surgery, a truly hallowed profession filled with pride, humility, gratitude, and satisfaction? Looking back at a career that spanned 37 years in the private practice of Vascular and General Surgery in West Palm Beach, Florida, I can genuinely say that it was a labor of love. Of course, I would never be foolish enough to state that every moment of every day was filled with joy and happiness. I recall many instances of sadness, regret, second-guessing, despair, and fatigue. However, I believe that anyone reflecting on my career would conclude that I have led a most worthy life.

Having become a voracious reader since my retirement from clinical practice, I understand that most want to avoid slogging through a long introduction. With that frame of reference, I will endeavor to keep this introduction short and focused. I will pose only two questions for you to consider while reading this book:

1. What was the "embryology" of this work? In other words, what pushed me to write this memoir, and exactly how did it develop?

2. Why will the information conveyed in this book be of value for generations of future physicians, young physicians just beginning in practice, and older physicians reflecting upon their careers? In other words, why should you read this book?

I will begin with the first question: How did this work come about? After I retired from my surgical practice in April 2013, I transitioned to an academic appointment as an Associate Professor of Surgery at Florida International University (FIU) Wertheim College of Medicine in Miami. In retrospect, I realized I missed this part of a surgical career, as until then, I was not fully involved with students and trainees or surrounded by a stimulating educational environment. As this type of opportunity was unavailable then in West Palm Beach, I commuted 87 miles (two hours) each way, five days a week, to arrive at the medical school by 8 AM. The opportunity to participate in the educational process and work directly with students was well worth the effort.

While there, one of the faculty members asked me if

I was willing to present a lecture to a group of pre-medical students from the Miami area who were taking a course at the medical school. I prepared a presentation entitled *"My 37-year Career in Surgical Practice."* While preparing this lecture, I reflected on my entire career, beginning with medical school at Cornell University Medical College (now known as Weill Cornell Medicine), my internship and residency in surgery at the Beth Israel Hospital-Harvard Medical School, additional senior and chief residency years at the Roosevelt Hospital (now known as Mount Sinai West) — Columbia University College of Physicians and Surgeons, and 37 years of clinical private practice. I was overjoyed to experience both interest and acclaim from the students. I appreciated their desire to contact me for further information and insights. I was delighted that my talk resonated with them and gave them a powerful, meaningful, and inspirational message.

℘ Virtual Shadowing

We now fast forward to September of 2020 and the COVID-19 pandemic. At the time, I was mentoring Ms Andrea Belen Serrano, who was then a pre-medical student at New York University (NYU), my undergraduate alma mater. She called me one day and asked if I would consider speaking as invited faculty as part of a pre-health virtual shadowing program in which she participated. As most of you know, one of the mandatory criteria in the medical school application process is participation in a "shadowing" experience, in which the applicant essentially follows the day-to-day activities of one or more practitioners on hospital rounds and in their offices.

With the pandemic in full bloom, this activity suddenly became impossible. To address this problem, Dr Raymond L. Fowler from the University of Texas Southwestern in Dallas and Ms Reagan Rosenberger, who was then a pre-medical student on a gap year from the University of North Texas, created a way for applicants to fulfill the shadowing requirement by participating in weekly virtual Zoom conferences with physicians and surgeons from various locations and with different areas of expertise. Ms Serrano had participated in these Zoom conferences for three months and raved about the overall experience. She told me that she thought (perhaps biased) that I, as her mentor, might be a superb contributor to this project. The next thing I knew, I was contacted, vetted, and asked to present a session on February 2, 2021. Ms Rosenberger contacted me about three weeks before this date, and I quickly decided to present the same talk that I had given at FIU. She said this would be perfect but asked if I could supplement the text with two clinical cases. Rather than emphasizing technical expertise, I drew on two experiences that highlighted the need for empathy, humility, giving back, professionalism, and sensitivity. These two cases effectively reflected the first part of my talk and broadly underscored the principles I was trying to demonstrate.

Tuesday, February 2, arrived, and, facing the computer on my desk in my home office, I began to speak. Although I had no prepared notes, I spoke freely using the PowerPoint slides as my guide. What was initially designed as a one-hour talk morphed into two hours and 20 minutes! Ms Rosenberger cautioned me to consider removing my contact information to avoid being inundated by calls from the participants after the talk. I (clearly naïvely) felt that this would not be a serious problem. I would consider it a privilege to speak with anyone, thinking that perhaps one or at most two students might choose to reach out. I had completed my talk by 9:30 PM, and by 10:15 PM, I began to receive text messages and emails from students asking to speak with me. Over the next few days, I was contacted by more than 60 students who had reached out for additional information. Even to this very day, I am occasionally contacted by some of the participants from this Zoom conference asking for advice. A link to my presentation is now available on YouTube as *"History and Insights into Surgery."**

Over the next few weeks, I was encouraged by surgical colleagues and friends to consider converting the information presented in this talk into a book. They convinced me that the information conveyed in this talk was compelling and meaningful and should not be permitted to rest unappreciated. Many of my colleagues remarked

---

* https://www.youtube.com/watch?v=Mbvo8gGT7Bo

that a book of this nature might become essential reading for all pre-medical and medical students, much like the 1921 classic *"Cope's Early Diagnosis of The Acute Abdomen,"* which was re-released in its 22nd Edition in March 2010 (revised by Dr William Silen). I am indebted to Ms Rosenberger, who generously volunteered to transcribe the audio presentation. I then reviewed and edited the text, adding the pertinent illustrations and images from my slide set.

❧ This Book Coming to Fruition

Before I knew it, we had reached the late fall/early winter of 2021, and I made a conscious effort to contact several major publishers. Much to my chagrin, there was no outpouring of interest in publishing my book. With that, the text more or less settled back onto a library shelf in my office where it rested! My book rested there until October 2023, when I was invited to be a guest faculty member at an International Symposium on Medicine and Surgery at The Universidad Privado Antenor Orrego in Trujillo, Peru. The organizing surgeon, Dr Jose Caballero, and I have been close colleagues and friends since July 2013, when I took 16 first-year medical students from FIU to this remote city in the northwest corner of Peru to work for two weeks in a regional hospital. I repeated this in 2014 and helped three of the practitioners at this facility become Fellows of The American College of Surgeons. When I arrived for the opening ceremonies for the conference, I quickly realized that the overwhelming majority of the 1500 attendees were medical students. The talks that I had prepared that focused on topics in surgery would be inappropriate for these students at this point in their education.

I asked the organizers if, instead of my originally scheduled talk, I could change the topic to the one addressed in my 2021 YouTube presentation. Although I speak Spanish reasonably well, my language skills were not quite good enough to present this two-hour talk. Ms Siorella Gonzales, a superb interpreter, came to my rescue and assisted with the presentation. We spent the entire evening working with the information technology personnel, who helped us to reformat the talk so that it could be given the following morning. I introduced Ms Gonzales in Spanish, and she proceeded with my presentation, word-for-word, also in Spanish! I was stunned when, upon completing the presentation, probably about 100 students from the auditorium stormed the stage. They all came up to me, thanking me, asking for pictures, shaking my hand, and hugging me. You would think I was a rock star! The faculty told me that the talk was so inspiring and emotional for these students, who were, of course, at the very earliest stages of their careers, so much so that its impact could not be measured. On the six-hour plane ride home, I once again considered trying to make this book happen.

So here we are. With the encouragement of a dear

colleague of more than 53 years, Dr Michael M. Meguid, MD, FACS (who provided a Foreword to this volume), and the youngest of my three sons (who are all Orthodox Jewish rabbis), Rabbi Dr Yosef Lynn, who is Dean of Students and a Senior Lecturer at Machon Yaakov in Jerusalem, this book has finally arrived.

So, what about my second question? Why does this book have value, and why should you read it? Once again, I beg your forgiveness if what I am about to say comes off as self-serving or bragging because that is certainly not my intent. It is with great humility that I, in a few short words, will attempt to convey its value to you, my current and future readers. I have been blessed to have stood upon the shoulders of giants, beginning with my undergraduate years at NYU, continuing at Cornell University Medical College, and culminating in my lifelong admiration for my most influential mentor, William Silen, MD, FACS, Emeritus Chair of Surgery at the Beth Israel Hospital, and The Johnson and Johnson Professor of Surgery at Harvard Medical School. Dr Silen unfortunately passed away in September of 2022 at the age of 95. Being at the graveside at his funeral in Boston and watching as he was lowered into the ground was a powerful experience and seemed to me to be the end of my youth and innocence. Having had the incredible privilege to rise within the ranks of academic surgical societies, notably as someone working in a fully non-university-based private practice and, most recently, serving as Second Vice-President of The American College of

Surgeons (2021-2022), I am fully aware of the changing paradigms in surgical education and the rising concerns about the maintenance of professionalism and ethics within our beloved calling.

Of even greater concern to me personally, many of our youngest students have begun to question events that they have witnessed within their chosen profession. Many are confused by the actions of some of their supposed role models and teachers that conflict with the essential moral principles embodied in the Hippocratic Oath.

My purpose in this short book is to highlight principles and practices that are both timeless and universal. These principles should never be violated, no matter what pressures you experience on any given day. In a time when physician "well-being" and "burnout" are of great concern, these principles will serve as an anchor and permit you to weather any imaginable storm.

Suppose you are reading this book because it was assigned as a prerequisite or part of a classroom syllabus. In that case, I sincerely hope you will come away with a feeling of freshness and pride in your chosen profession and that you will ultimately be grateful to your teachers and mentors who insisted on this. If you are reading this at the twilight of a long and honorable career, I hope you will feel that you stayed true to the course and can feel validated and proud of your accomplishments.

Now, we will proceed with my story without any further ado.

CHAPTER ONE

It's Not About Me

Where You Fit In

I WANT TO REPEAT and emphasize this point: *It's not about me.*

This book is really about you. My goal is to provide you with insight and information that I needed but didn't have available to me when I was finishing undergraduate study and considering a career in medicine.

No one in my family was a physician. No one in my family had even finished college, and no one had the kind of insight and advice that I might have benefited from at the time. So, I more or less winged it, and it turned out okay. I'm fairly proud and pleased with what I've achieved and where I am at this point in my life. But again, this is not about me. This is about conveying to you all what a medical career is about. Although surgery has been my vocation, I believe that my insights and personal views apply to the role of the physician and the practice of medicine in general. I genuinely think that it is essential to remain focused and keep your "antennae" up as you accumulate decades of experiences, high points, low points, and successes and failures, as well as periods of calm and turmoil so that one day you too will be able to reflect on a whole career and your entire life.

Let me begin with a bit of background about myself. I grew up in Long Island, New York, with one sister and two working parents in what was then considered a lower-middle-class home. Nonetheless, I graduated Phi Beta Kappa in 1967 from New York University (NYU) Washington Square College of Arts and Sciences. I lived at home and commuted by bus and subway to classes in the city every day of my undergraduate career. Fortunately, I was accepted to Cornell University Medical College (now known as Weill Cornell Medicine), where I had an incredible four years. Then, I began my surgical training at Harvard University at the Beth Israel Hospital in Boston under the direction of Dr William Silen, who you will hear more about later. I then continued my training in New York at the Roosevelt Hospital of Columbia University College of Physicians and Surgeons. To this day, I am not exactly sure why I decided to begin my private surgical practice in West Palm Beach, Florida, but I am here, and I have no regrets.

☙ Attitude ❧

"The longer I live, the more I realize the impact of attitude on life. Attitude, to me, is more important than facts.

It is more important than the past, the education, the money, than circumstances, than failure, than successes, than what other people think or say or do. It is more important than appearance, giftedness or skill. It will make or break a company... a church... a home.

The remarkable thing is we have a choice everyday regarding the attitude we will embrace for that day.

We cannot change our past... we cannot change the fact that people will act in a certain way. We cannot change the inevitable.

The only thing we can do is play on the one string we have, and that is our attitude.

I am convinced that life is 10% what happens to me and 90% of how I react to it. And so it is with you... we are in charge of our attitudes."

— Charles R. Swindoll

Before we begin our journey, I think it would help if we all reflected for a few moments on the text of the poem "Attitude," written by Charles Swindoll, an evangelical Christian pastor, author, educator, and radio personality. In a few brief lines, Mr. Swindoll summarized what, in my mind, life is all about. Your life will not end after one, two, or four years out of medical school. Your attitude and outlook will be the force that molds your career and your future.

CHAPTER TWO

There Will Always Be New Challenges

꧁ Challenges I Faced during My Surgical Career

MY 37-YEAR CAREER in surgery did not end the day I finished medical school or my training. It had just begun.

I first think of staplers when I think of everything that changed and evolved over nearly forty years in surgical practice. You might ask, what was so important about this? For hundreds of years, before the late 1960s and early 1970s, wounds were closed in the operating room by actual sewing with sutures (i.e., thread) and needles operated by a pair of highly skilled hands. Then, suddenly, this entire revolution came about. Mechanical stapling could now be used to replace sewing with your hands. Having trained during the period in which staplers were evolving, this sudden change was anxiety-provoking. Although I had minimal experience with these devices,

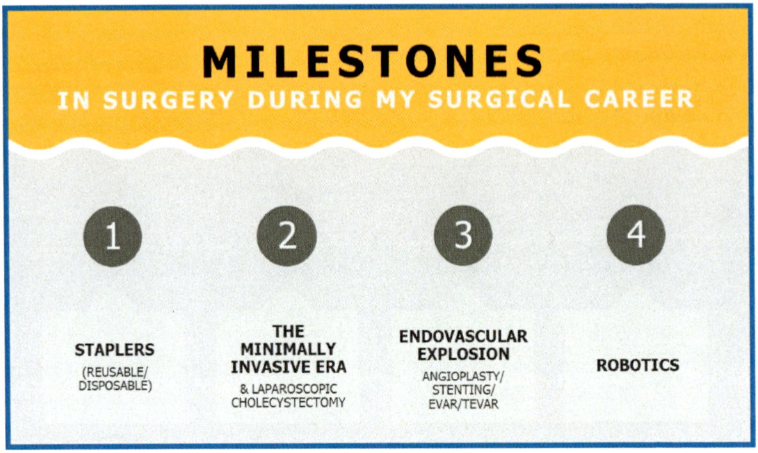

they seemed to be taking over how anastomoses (i.e., techniques for putting things together) were performed.

I rose to the challenge and mastered this new technique, as did all of my colleagues who were my age at the time. Suddenly, at around 1990, a second challenge arose. Remember, I had been in practice for 14 years at that time. I had probably performed well over a thousand standard cholecystectomies (i.e., gall bladder removals). This complex and invasive procedure, which was more or less the "bread and butter" of general surgical practice, involved an abdominal incision and removal of the diseased organ from just below the liver. Then, seemingly overnight, a video from a small community hospital in Tennessee demonstrated how to remove the gallbladder through a minor incision in the navel plus three small probes. Suddenly, this became the new gold standard.

As you can see, it wasn't just a matter of adapting

what I had done for 14 years with added nuance; this procedure was highly distant from anything I had ever seen, heard of, read, or experienced. So here I am, in my mid-40s and 14 years into practice, and seemingly overnight, patients want to have their gallbladders removed in this new way. How would we older surgeons learn how to do this *right now*? Training in the new procedure was offered as a mini-course that took place over two weekend days (if you were lucky enough to secure a spot). This was followed by some didactics by the pioneers of this methodology. You successfully performed the procedure on a pig, and then you were done! This is different from how things should have been, but that's how it was back then. Fortunately, new surgical procedures are now introduced in a more thorough manner.

If that wasn't a sufficient boost to my overall anxiety levels, we can now consider the third challenge. I was trained as both a vascular surgeon and a general surgeon. Early on, I decided to continue to perform both vascular and general surgery in my practice because I liked and was proficient at both types of procedures. However, I was committed to performing only those procedures where my skills remained "state of the art." In ~1999/2000, the United States Food and Drug Administration (the FDA) approved the first endovascular aortic stent graft that could be used to repair aneurysms. Before these stent grafts were available, repair of an aortic aneurysm involved a major abdominal incision; the graft was sewn in place, and the aneurysm was then excluded. I had mastered this very invasive operation and performed it hundreds of times. Suddenly, however, this major operation could now be done by creating a small puncture in the groin and by repairing the aneurysm with wires and catheters threaded through the arteries. The patients needed no invasive abdominal incisions and could be discharged back home in one or two days. This was a significant change as previously, patients typically stayed in the hospital for seven to ten days (initially in the ICU for 2-3 days), and this was the procedure if everything went perfectly!

If you had told me after I had completed my training that a procedure such as this would become the "gold standard," I would have thought you were imagining things! You must remember, I was in a solo practice. I had no connections to a university program where I would have had the opportunity to learn how to do these new procedures from younger colleagues with more recent training. Ultimately, I decided to take time off from my surgical practice and travel around the country to master these new techniques.

Finally, we come to the fourth challenge. Robotic surgery became available (FDA approved) in ~2004 or 2005. I realized early on that these techniques were about to become a major force in modern surgery and that I needed to gain expertise in using this platform.

I then quickly got involved in robotic abdominal surgery and only picked out robotic procedures that could benefit from the implementation—not just because it was easier or marketable.

As you reflect on my journey through these challenges in my surgical career, remember that resilience and adaptability are critical traits for anyone pursuing a long and fulfilling path, whether in medicine or any other field. Each advancement I encountered—from staplers to laparoscopic cholecystectomy to endovascular stenting—was daunting and disruptive and required me to completely rethink my approach to surgery. But rather than being discouraged, I leaned into the challenge and committed to learning, even when it meant starting over or taking time away to retrain.

Life, like a career in surgery, will continuously present you with challenges. Some may be technical, while others are personal, yet all require that same willingness to adapt, grow, and persevere. Know that setbacks and challenges don't signify defeat; they are simply part of the process. The true mark of progress isn't the absence of obstacles but the courage to face them with an open mind and an enduring commitment to learn. Embrace each change as an opportunity because, through these trials, you'll build your skills and resilience, preparing you for a lifetime of growth.

CHAPTER THREE

The Learning Never Ends

"The brighter you are, the more you have to learn."

— Don Herold (July 9, 1889 - June 1, 1966)
American humorist, writer, illustrator

ꕤ Double-Edged Sword: Intellectually stimulating yet anxiety provoking, but always challenging and gratifying

WHAT DOES THIS REALLY MEAN? Every single student enrolled in medical school is bright. Every medical student has a high IQ, has done well in school, and is a proven learner. So, the brighter you are, the more you have to learn. This is, of course, a double-edged sword. Although learning new things can be intellectually stimulating, a job that requires you to apply new knowledge not once but again and again can often be anxiety-provoking. Here you are, feeling comfortable with your skills and abilities and at the point where you can do certain things almost blindfolded. Suddenly, you find yourself back at the starting line in your mid-40s and 50s, and someone who is 30 years old has new and vital skills that exceed yours. While this is of course anxiety-provoking, remember to meet the challenge head-on. It will also be gratifying in the end.

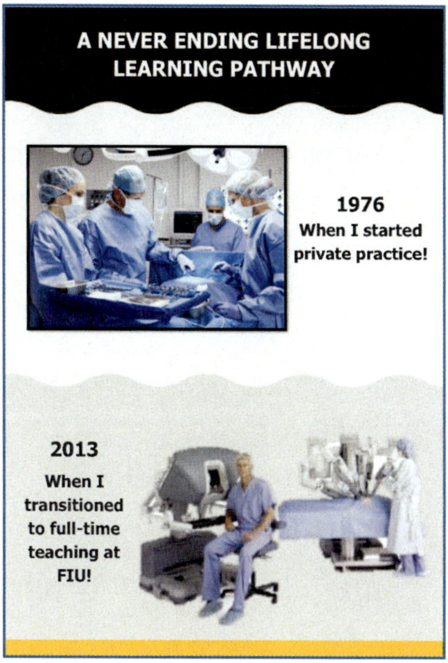

☙ A Never-Ending Lifelong Learning Pathway: Then and now

At 20 or 21, it is difficult, if not impossible, to think about what you might be doing when you're 67 (or 72 or 73). However, it's essential to recognize that your chosen career is part of a lifelong, never-ending learning pathway. The picture above is that of an operating room circa 1976 when I began my private practice. Shown here is a surgeon, a surgical assistant, an anesthesiologist, a scrub tech, and all of the instruments needed to perform an open operation, which are laid out on the table in front. In 2013, when I transitioned to full-time teaching at FIU, you, suddenly were no longer standing next to the patient. Instead, you sat at a console and performed the robotic operation while glued to the camera and the devices that permitted you to control the surgical robot. Please note: the robot doesn't do the operation (you do!!); however, it carries out instructions and commands that permit it to do what you want. The robot responds to your commands (typically small wrist motions). You are not standing near the operating table or wearing an operating gown. Who would have believed this would be an everyday reality in 1976?

Continued Lifelong Learning

Similar changes have been introduced in the world of vascular surgery. An aortic aneurysm, which is typically a large, weak blister in the wall of the aorta, is a life-threatening condition and is associated with significant morbidity and mortality. The world-renowned physicist Albert Einstein died from a ruptured aneurysm, as did actors George C. Scott and Lucille Ball.

In these earlier years, an aortic aneurysm was repaired using a method pioneered by Michael DeBakey and Denton Cooley in Houston, Texas. A major incision was made in the abdomen that extended from the xiphoid to the pubis. The aorta was exposed, and all the major components were identified and isolated. The aneurysm was opened, and a graft was sewn to replace the damaged region. Patients were monitored for several days in the intensive care unit, and if no complications ensued, they were sent home to recover after seven to ten days. Now, and in 2013, the entire procedure was performed using catheters that were sent up through the arteries that were introduced by a small puncture in the groin. The graft is inserted and placed appropriately via a fluoroscopically-guided controlled catheter. The patient leaves the procedure suite with two small bandages covering the wound in the groin. The patient typically sits up that evening on a regular diet and is discharged the following day. When I was in training, this possibility was beyond my wildest imagination.

❧ Changes in My Career vs Those that Came Before Me

When my teachers finished their careers, from 1948 to 1980, they experienced a very different world of medicine.

When I entered surgical training in 1971, I was mentored by some surgeons who were nearing the end of their careers. Most had completed their training in or around 1948, practiced for thirty to forty years, and retired in 1980. In my naïve view at the time, they were fortunate because nothing really changed from the technology standpoint. For example, an anastomosis of two ends of the colon was performed in 1980, pretty much exactly as it had been in 1948, and they didn't have to worry about using staplers. Similarly, a gallbladder excision was performed more or less identically in 1948 and 1980; laparoscopic surgery had not yet emerged into the mainstream. I'm not saying they didn't have to learn anything; however, from a technical standpoint, they didn't find themselves awake at night worrying about how to perform their very first laparoscopic appendectomy at fifty-plus years of age. The significant advances seen during my predecessors' decades included the introduction of antibiotics, intensive care units, new advances in preoperative and postoperative care, and anesthesia methods. These changes did not significantly impact the actual technical performance of routine surgical procedures.

CHAPTER FOUR

A Good Mentor Is Everything

☙ I Owe It All to My Mentor – William Silen, MD, FACS

I BELIEVE WITH EVERY bone in my body that I owe my successes in my surgical career to my mentor, Dr William Silen. Dr Silen was the Johnson & Johnson Professor of Surgery at Harvard Medical School and Chairman of the Department of Surgery at Beth Israel Hospital in Boston. He came to Harvard in 1967 from the University of California San Francisco, where he proceeded to revolutionize the world of surgery at

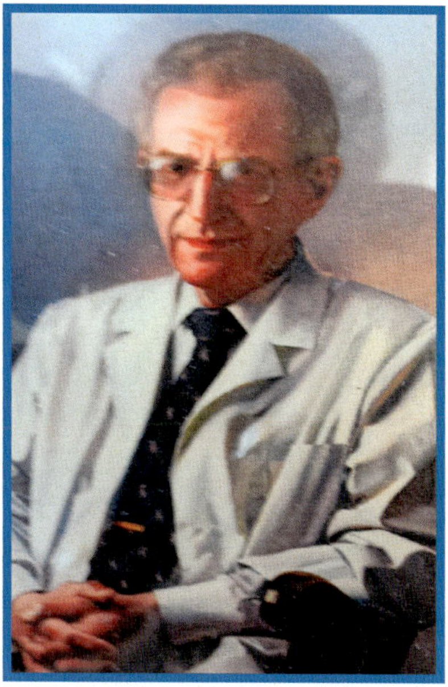

Willam Silen, MD, FACS

Beth Israel/Harvard. Since 1974, Dr Silen had been the sole editor of *Cope's Early Diagnosis of the Acute Abdomen,* which was and remains the classic treatise in our field.

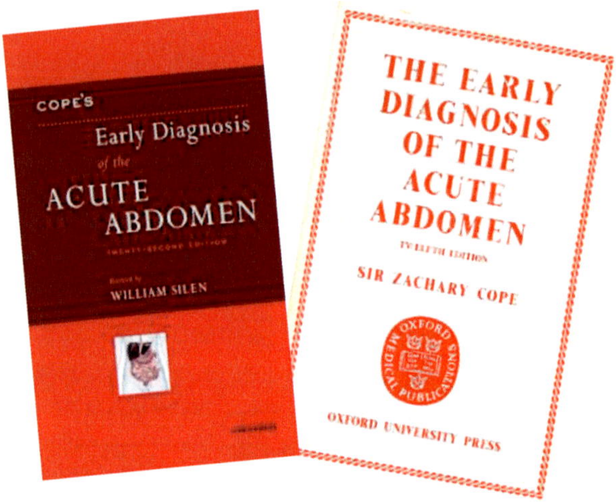

A very long time ago, before computed tomography (CT), magnetic resonance imaging (MRI), and ultrasound technology, physicians came up with diagnoses based on the patient's history and a physical exam. We had only some limited laboratory data such as blood count, blood chemistries, urine analysis, and blood cultures, as well as very primitive radiographic procedures such as plain films, fluoroscopic studies in GI areas, and limited angiography. Dr Zachary Cope (1881-1974), who was a surgeon in England, felt that people were dying unnecessarily due to either failure to diagnose (still the number one factor underlying medical litigation) or inappropriate treatment. To address this concern, he wrote a book entitled, *The Early Diagnosis of the Acute Abdomen*. What is an "acute" abdomen, you might ask? Essentially, this means, "I don't know what the patient has going on intra-abdominally, but he or she will die without an immediate operation." This is more or less what an acute abdomen meant in 1921, and it means pretty much the same thing today. In other words, you don't need to know exactly what is going on internally; you only need to get the patient into the operating room so that you can diagnose and fix the problem right now. Otherwise, the patient is likely to die!

Furthermore, it is equally essential to ensure that you are not taking someone to the operating room who does not need to undergo an invasive procedure. Only the surgeons made this decision; of course, they had to visit the hospital to see the patient. Surgeons did not diagnose patients over the phone and did not say, *"Let me know what the CT scan shows before I come in."* You, the surgeon, had to come in, and you alone had to make that decision.

When Dr Cope died in 1974, the book was probably in its 20th edition as he changed it over the years to reflect progress, particularly in diagnostic modalities. Dr Silen, at the time of his passing in 2022 at 95 years of age, had been the only other physician to serve as editor of this important book. Cope's family knew of Dr Silen and understood that he would continue to exemplify these crucial principles of patient care. When I retired from clinical private practice in 2013, I became an Associate

Professor of Surgery at the new medical school that had opened at FIU in Miami. I brought this book back into the curriculum and made it required reading for third-year surgical clerkship didactic sessions. While some of the younger students thought I was old-fashioned because they believed that everything they needed to know could be determined by CT scan or MRI, I insisted, and now it's part of the curriculum.

℘ The Value of Bedside Skills In a Technological Era

I'm sure many board-certified emergency room physicians hesitate before calling in a surgeon. Although things are a bit different in a university department, nobody wants to be on call in private practice, and certainly no one wants to come in off-hours. Thus, when the emergency room physician calls and says, "I need you," some colleagues would respond, "What does the CT scan show?" If the CT scan was normal, he or she might refuse to come in.

It is also interesting to note that, in the early 1970s, a surgeon who did not remove normal appendices (typically in about 10% of cases) was considered not operating often enough. Today, if you take out a normal appendix, you might find yourself answering to a quality-assessment committee. Why the change? This is because everyone gets a CT scan. Does every patient actually need a CT scan? Probably not. Many patients who present with classic acute appendicitis could be taken to the operating room immediately and spared the delay and the radiation exposure. Importantly, this would also reduce the unnecessary costs added to an already overburdened healthcare system, but the horse is already out of the barn!

Bedside assessment is a critical and fundamental skill. When I became a faculty member in 2013, I saw how Observed Structured Clinical Examinations (OSCEs) were performed. These are important tests used to ensure that students are skilled in physical diagnosis. The examiners essentially went through a checklist. Did the student know how to percuss? If yes, they checked off the box. Did the student palpate? If yes, again, check off the box. Even when all the boxes were checked, very few students could use these skills to diagnose anything; these skills were considered mainly unimportant relics.

In reality, nothing could be further from the truth. When I transitioned to full-time academics, I took 16 first-year medical students to spend two weeks in Trujillo, a small town in Northern Peru, nine hours from Lima by bus. CT and MRI scanners were not readily available there. Suddenly, the students needed to diagnose patients using the same skills Dr Cope and Dr Silen used. To students who think, "Well, I don't need all this," I would say, you really never know. As recently as 2005, when Hurricane Katrina ripped through New Orleans, Louisiana State University, Tulane, and Charity Hospitals were wiped out for a full 10 days. There was no electricity and no CT scans, and yet people developed bowel obstructions, perforations, and appendicitis just the same. Physicians needed to diagnose these conditions based on skills that, unfortunately, are perceived as old-fashioned and unnecessary by many students in this younger generation. This is simply not true. I'm old-fashioned, and I don't apologize for that.

CHAPTER FIVE

The Pursuit of Excellence

℘ A Tribute to Dr William Silen: A few vignettes

WHEN I ARRIVED at Harvard, I had just completed what might be considered classical training at Cornell University Medical College. I had heard stories about Dr Silen, but I had no idea what I would encounter. The first thing to know is, when you were on his service, you needed to be at the hospital at 3:00 AM to make rounds on his patients because, believe it or not, Dr Silen, the esteemed Johnson & Johnson Professor of Surgery at Harvard, arrived each day at 5:00 AM. He made rounds with his team, had breakfast, and went to the operating room. His day began this way because he had so many obligations as a Department Chairman and a faculty member at Harvard Medical School that this was the only time that he had to sit at the patient's bedside to talk and examine the patient, as opposed to just breezing by and asking us *"How's everything boys?"* I'm ashamed to say that I thought he was nuts at the time! He went on and on about so many details. None of the great surgeons I trained with in New York acted like this. Unfortunately, although I am beyond thankful that I ultimately learned what he taught, I didn't appreciate his greatness until after I had left his tutelage.

℘ Classic Dr Silen Quotations

Although Dr Silen had millions of quotations, these three stand out.

> "There is no such thing as minor surgery, only minor surgeons."

Take a moment to reflect on this. What was he really saying? His message was that, while a small boil, minor abscess, or slight hernia may seem trivial to you, the patient isn't concerned with your expertise in major procedures. The patient cares only about what this issue means for them personally and how you will address it.

> "There are no mysteries in medicine, only mysterious doctors."

What does this mean? Sometimes, things simply don't go as planned. An inexperienced physician might say, "I don't know what happened—it was a mystery." But, in truth, it wasn't a mystery; the answer was right there—you just didn't see it. As a surgeon, you must learn to see everything.

Finally, despite the common stereotype that surgeons prefer action over thought, Dr. Silen believed that...

"Surgeons should be internists that operate."

Dr Silen was a member of the Editorial Board of the *New England Journal of Medicine*, the pre-eminent medical, non-surgical journal in the United States. He was President of the American Gastroenterological Association, whose members are primarily medical gastroenterologists. The 1997 Surgical Forum of The American College of Surgeons Clinical Congress was dedicated to him. Clearly, the world knows that Dr Silen was a respected scholar and highly skilled surgeon.

Upon arriving at Harvard, I received a "survival manual." This was a 15-page typewritten, single-spaced document that included just about all of Dr Silen's specific activities and expectations. This manual was created by a resident who preceded me and simply could not abide by Dr Silen and his strict ways. When Dr Silen finally had enough of this, he transferred this resident to his gastric physiology laboratory, but at the same time, insisted that he needed to generate a written guide so that future residents would know exactly what to expect.

I still have the original manual in my files (see Appendix A)!

Early Realizations

3 Things I Wish I'd Realized Earlier

1. "Youth is wasted on youth."
2. "When you are amongst the forest you can't see over the trees."
3. "The older you get, the smarter your parents and teachers become."

These are the three things that I wish I had realized when I was a younger man. As a surgical resident at Harvard, my fellow Intern and I would wander out into the hall while on rounds with Dr Silen. I knew nothing, and my fellow intern knew nothing, yet here we were chatting and criticizing him. We were hanging out, just killing time while he was going on and on at the bedside when, all of a sudden, he noticed me and called out, *"Lynn, the pearls are in here,"* meaning that the wisdom I needed was there with him at the bedside, not out in the hall.

Fortunately, learning is lifelong. At some point, if we're lucky, we begin to realize what we were exposed to and what's happening around us. It would be great if we understood this from the start, but we all learn as we go. This is true for marriage, parenting, and everything else.

☙ Presidential Address: 5 values

Dr Carlos Pellegrini was the Chair of Surgery for many years at the University of Washington, Seattle. He was also the first Latin American President of the American College of Surgeons. He became the President of this organization in 2013, the 100th anniversary of the American College of Surgeons, initially founded in 1913. In his presidential address, Dr Pelligrini spoke about the five essential values everyone in our profession needs to uphold.

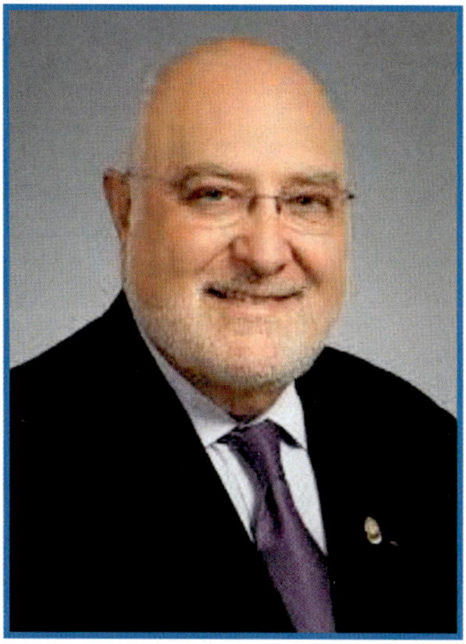

Dr Carlos Pellegrini, MD, FACS
President,
American College of Surgeons
2013-2014

I was in the audience then and have always remembered his words. At the time, Dr Pelligrini was speaking to the new initiates as Fellows of the American College of Surgeons (FACS). After all the training, including medical school, residency, fellowship, and board certification, Dr Pelligrini chose to speak to them about *"Professionalism, Excellence, Innovation, Introspection, and Inclusion."* I don't think I need to say more about those five points because they remain as relevant today as they were just ten years ago. Unfortunately, many of you just entering the profession may encounter colleagues who do not behave professionally. You may not be able to do anything about it, but you must register your observations and ensure you do not emulate these colleagues.

℘ Five Values to Guide ☙ Professional Practice

1. Professionalism
2. Excellence
3. Innovation
4. Introspection
5. Inclusion

℘ The Importance of Doing What Is Right, Even When It Is Against the Status Quo

> "If you want to make enemies, try to change something."

Although this point has been made by many people and in many situations, the quote is attributed to Woodrow Wilson, the 28th President of the United States. President Wilson was known for many things, including his unsuccessful efforts to establish the League of Nations. My message to you is that if you see and experience things that are not right during your career, you should not remain silent. While you may not choose to scream and yell, you might identify appropriate channels for clarification, communication, and correction. You need to speak up rather than just look the other way.

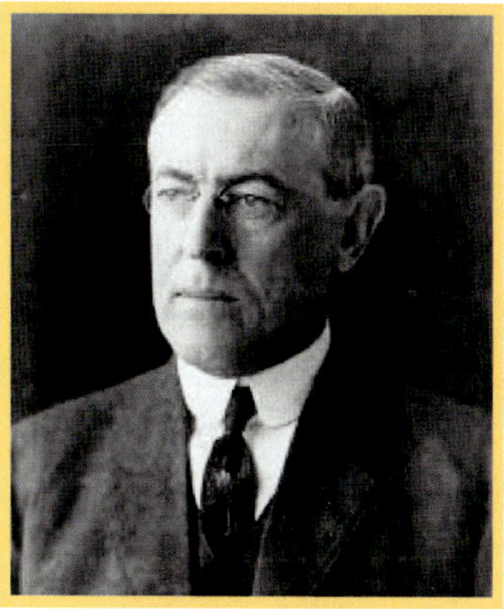

Woodrow Wilson, 28th President of the United States

In 1889, brothers Charles and William Mayo, opened a medical clinic in the middle of a cornfield in Rochester, MN. Among their most famous quotes:

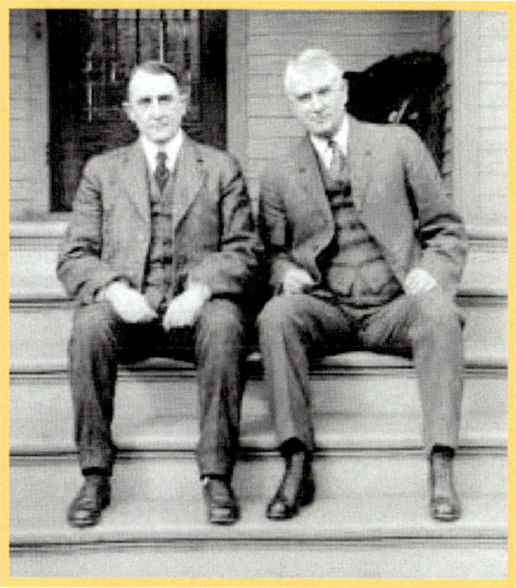

Charles and William Mayo, Medical Pioneers

"Having a person's life in your hands is an awesome responsibility."

Please remember this. No matter how difficult the situation, no matter how disgruntled, frustrated, or beaten down you may be, remember that having a person's life in your hands is a profound responsibility!

The Qualities of a Successful Surgeon – John Morton

Dr John Morton, Professor of Surgery at Strong Memorial Hospital of the University of Rochester, published a brief essay in the *Archives of Surgery* entitled *"The Qualities of a Successful Surgeon."* In this essay, Dr Morton noted that he had been asked to speak at the funeral service of a very close friend who was also a surgeon. In preparing his remarks, he began to think more about this man and came up with a list of ten characteristics embodied by his late friend. Some of these characteristics are more or less intuitive, such as *a warm personality*. In other words, you need to be a person. You cannot come into an examination room acting "holier than thou," standing in your starched white coat and speaking to your patients. You need to be a human being.

Another value, *intelligence*, is also a "no-brainer." Likewise, having *an ethical approach* should also be apparent. You should always behave ethically. When you find yourself caught between what the insurance company wants, what the hospital wants, or what the financial controller wants, you must be able to speak up and do the right thing. Number four, *humility*, is also essential. That does not mean a surgeon should be timid; I would want my surgeon to be humble enough and have enough self-confidence to reach out for help if he or she needs it. I'm proud to say that I did just this when I needed to. I have never hesitated to call out to a colleague, even if he confirmed my choices at the end of the day. I felt better for doing this. Likewise, all surgeons must have *courage*, meaning the courage of their convictions.

Finally, surgeons must engage in *self-analysis*. Don't beat yourself over the head to a point where you can no longer function. However, if something is amiss, you cannot say "next case" and move on as though nothing has happened.

This book isn't about my journey alone; it's about you and the insights I wish I'd had when I started in medicine. I came from a family without doctors or college graduates, and my path involved navigating challenges and new skills—like stapling, laparoscopic cholecystectomy, and robotic surgery—all requiring adaptability. The heart of this journey lies in resilience, self-reflection, and a willingness to learn continuously. As Charles Swindoll said, attitude shapes not just our day but our careers. In medicine, staying open to growth and embodying qualities like humility, ethics, and courage is crucial for long-term success and fulfillment.

CHAPTER SIX

Selected Questions and Answers

WITH THAT BACKGROUND IN MIND, let's delve into some questions that many aspiring medical professionals have. From my unconventional journey to medical school to the future of surgery, I'll address common questions that reflect both personal experiences and broader trends in the field. This discussion will provide valuable insights into navigating your career path and adapting to the evolving landscape of medicine.

Q. *You mentioned that none of your family members were physicians or healthcare professionals. How did that impact your decision to go to medical school?*

A. Growing up, being a doctor was probably the farthest thing from my mind. I did well in school, but I didn't even like science. This was the early 1960s, and I wanted to quit school and go on tour with our band. I played drums, and we were actually pretty good! We made a few records that played on some radio shows. I even performed one evening with the legendary Frankie Valli and The Four Seasons when their drummer was nowhere to be found. Our band, The Ideals, had been the opening act for The Four Seasons. Needless to say, my parents were not on board with this.

I was also reasonably talented at drawing and painting, and my mother insisted that I attend art school one afternoon a week (which I wouldn't say I liked because all my friends were out playing ball at the time). I went to college thinking I would combine art and mathematics and perhaps be an architect. Nonetheless, on the first day of college in 1963, I registered as a pre-medical student. I've done a lot of soul-searching about this over the past sixty years. Maybe this was because my grandmother, with whom I was very close, was living with us while dying from cancer.

Or maybe (finally!!), I did it to please my parents. I must admit that I was not your standard "good student." My mother was always perplexed about "what to do with me" because I was perpetually misbehaving–not in any terrible way, but I was mischievous and kind of a "wise guy." At the same time, my father was very strict. All I ever heard from him was that I wouldn't amount to anything. Maybe I chose pre-med because, after all, what does every Jewish mother and father want? "My son, the doctor!" They never said this to me outright, but subconsciously, perhaps this is why I registered as a pre-medical student. Of course, the rest is history!

Q. *How do you think the field of surgery will change over the next decade?*

A. There is no question in my mind that things will continue to change. First, there will be less and less need for surgery; this is already happening for several well-known disease processes. Operations that I learned and performed hundreds of times as a resident-in-training simply no longer exist. Perhaps the best example of this is surgery for gastric ulceration. In earlier times, one of the most common indications for surgery was bleeding in the upper gastrointestinal tract secondary to ulcer disease. This procedure has essentially disappeared from the face of the earth because of the availability of Prilosec and Zantac. I don't care if you're the busiest surgeon in the world; you're lucky if you do maybe three or four procedures for non-malignant gastric disease in an entire year.

Q. *Does anyone still receive training in Billroth procedures (i.e., gastroduodenostomies or gastrojejunostomies)?*

A. While medical therapies have largely eliminated the need for these procedures, there will always be occasional patients who need them. I'm sad to say that the only surgeons capable of performing these procedures are older and likely to be retired or retiring. So, although we will all experience even greater progress over time, there will always be patients who might benefit from this approach; for example, injuries due to trauma are never going to disappear. Likewise, acute appendicitis is never going to go away. However, I think that these surgical procedures will become less and less frequent, and those that remain will be minimally invasive and will use nanotechnology-based tools.

Q. *Although many things have changed, and here I'm thinking particularly about devices intended to limit trauma and increase safety, such as seatbelts, how has the availability and use of these devices changed surgical practice?*

A. When medical students ask me for advice on choosing a specialty, I tell them to think about what they would be doing today and whether their practice is likely to be the same in years to come.

As we have discussed, operative open surgery is rapidly disappearing. So, if you're driven by the possibility of performing extensive incisions and open surgery, you may find yourself disappointed in the long and even in the short run. You need to look at the medical/surgical specialties and try to determine what specific practice will be like 15, 20, and even 30 years from now. Although organ transplantation is likely to continue and will most likely require open surgery, at least in the short term, this is not the case for all procedures. For example, the number of open cardiac procedures has diminished astronomically since the introduction of angioplasty and statins. If you're looking at the big picture, i.e., "What am I going do for the next 40 years," some fields will always be there (thinking, Psychiatry, and Pathology). Still, as a third-year medical student, you must consider what things are like today and what you might be doing at age fifty.

CHAPTER SEVEN

Case Studies

The following are two important case studies from my long career. Please consider deeply the meaning and implications of each vignette.

꩜ ***Case #1: In for a surprise*** ꩜

To quote my mentor, Dr Silen, "There are no minor surgeries, only minor surgeons." You will see why this quote is directly relevant to this case.

Mr Z was a 60-plus-year-old African American male who presented to my office on a clinic day with a chief complaint of having a lump in his neck. As you can see, the mass was quite large. I was certainly surprised to find out about this. I had never seen anything like this before, and neither had the two medical students who accompanied me to the clinic on that day.

Mr Z told me he first noticed a small lump around ten years ago. When he showed it to his doctor, he was told to leave it alone because "it's not bothering you" and "it's nothing." Over the years, the lump continued to enlarge. Although he sought medical attention, his concerns were routinely dismissed, and he became convinced that nothing could be done. Finally, somebody referred him to me because (unlike many of my local colleagues) I accepted Medicaid, a government program that provides healthcare coverage for low-income individuals.

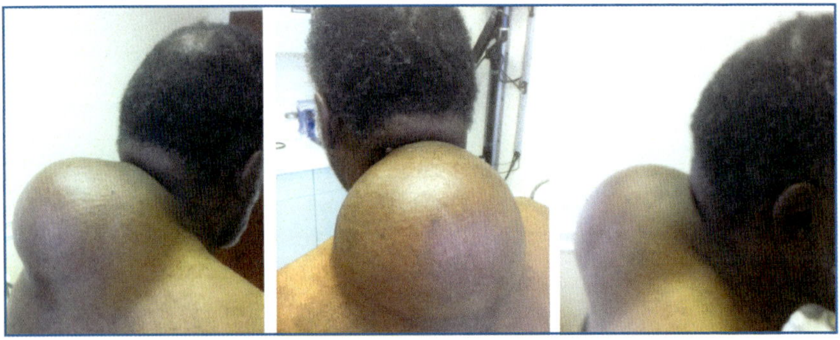

A 60-plus-year-old African American male presented with a large lump on the back of his neck.

Fortunately, the MRI scan that I ordered revealed that the mass was not impinging on the spinal canal, leading me to believe that I could achieve satisfactory results for this patient. I told Mr Z that I could remove the mass but that this would not be minor surgery and would take a few hours. It bothered me immensely that Mr Z had been tossed about, most likely because of his insurance status and the fact that lesions such as this are typically considered *"uninteresting."*

Also of note, Mr Z told me that he was a Jehovah's Witness and that he would refuse any blood transfusions. Although this was a sizable mass and substantial blood loss was, of course, a possibility, I told him that I would do the best that I could.

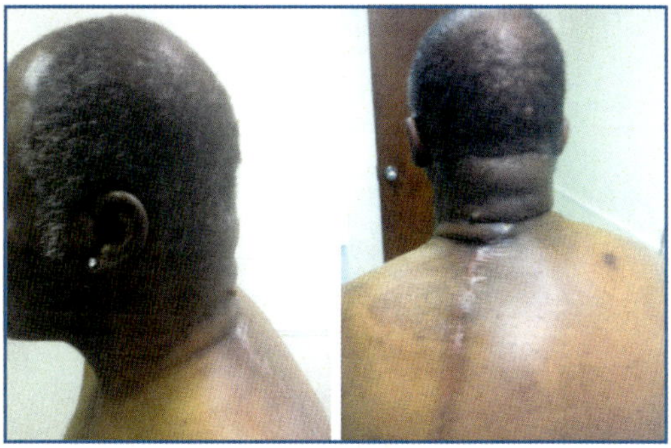

A large fatty lipoma with no malignant features was removed.

The three-hour-long procedure was performed with the patient in a prone position. At the first postoperative visit, when the bandages and drains were removed, Mr Z looked into the mirror and began to cry. On the final visit, we hugged each other, and I wished him well.

This is, of course, a straightforward case that involved no special procedures or technical finesse. However, it is important to recognize that this man had been passed around and largely dismissed. The system failed him. Although his care did not involve an endovascular aortic aneurysm, a carotid endarterectomy, or liver resection (i.e., complex procedures that might be of interest to a surgeon), to him, this was the most critical thing in the world. No dollar value can be assigned to being able to do right by Mr Z and having had the privilege of caring for this man.

Case #2: A truly emotional journey

Although the case I am about to present features a procedure known as carotid endarterectomy, the story unfolding is really about our relationships with the patients and families who have come to us for care, and not just the procedure.

The first book, *Doctors Cry, Too*, was written by Dr Boehm in the late 1990s for the lay public. He also wrote a second book two or three years later, *Building Patient/Doctor Trust*.

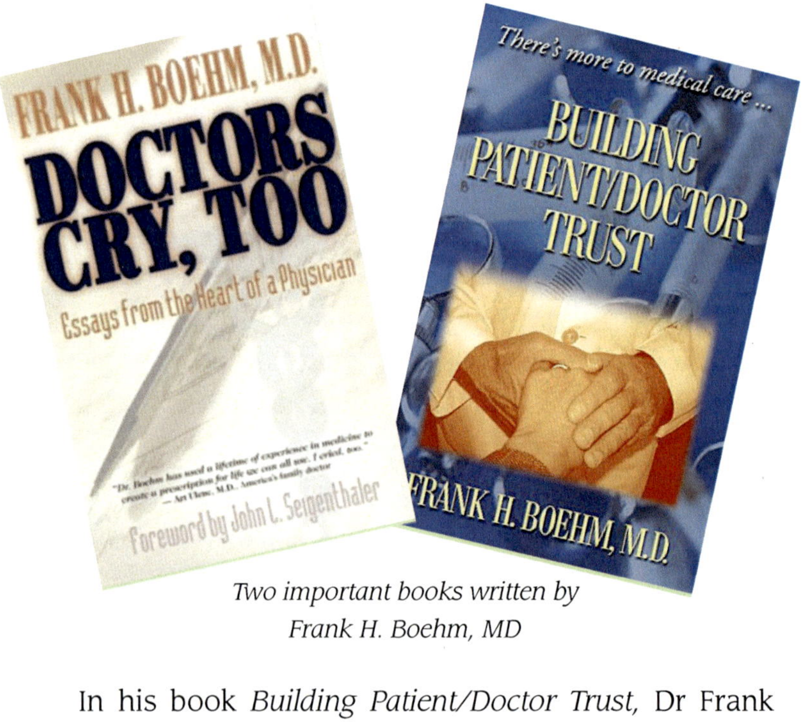

Two important books written by Frank H. Boehm, MD

In his book *Building Patient/Doctor Trust,* Dr Frank Boehm examines health care and its current functioning.

He shares his experiences and opinions about the medical and political sides of medicine. He points out that the traditional relationship between patients and doctors—where decisions focus on the patient's needs—has changed because of modern managed-care systems.

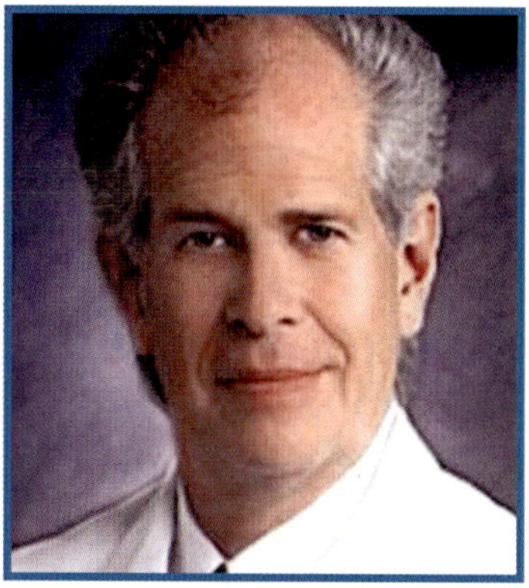

Dr Frank Boehm

Dr Boehm believes good medical care is about more than treating health problems. It's also about building trust between patients and doctors. He says doctors must listen carefully and understand how a patient's personal life affects their health. At the same time, patients should have meaningful conversations with their doctors to help strengthen the bond between patients and doctors.

Dr Boehm was a Professor of Obstetrics and Gynecology, a former Director of High-Risk Maternal-Fetal Medicine, and the former Chair of the Ethics Committee at Vanderbilt University. His book, *Doctors Cry, Too*, was first published in 2001, shortly after the famous 1999 paper from the Institute of Medicine entitled *To Err is Human,* which acknowledged the hundreds of thousands of deaths and complications that occurred in hospitals yearly due to medical error. At that time, the public's perception of doctors was deteriorating rapidly. Many believed doctors cared only about money and lifestyle and that the days of the presumably more compassionate doctors of the 1950s were gone forever. Dr Boehm wanted to write this book to let the lay public know this was not the case.

I met Dr Boehm in Nashville shortly after he published this book. Many years later, when I was The President of the Florida Chapter of the American College of Surgeons, I asked Dr Boehm to speak at our four-day symposium. I remember distinctly that many tears were shed by the surgeons in the audience.

With this as an introduction, Case #2 involves a man in his late 70s who was vacationing in Florida and was admitted to the hospital with a diagnosis of repetitive strokes, known as crescendo transient ischemic attacks (TIAs), due to severe high-grade carotid blockage. The attending physician and neurologist believed this condition needed to be addressed immediately. (Note that this was before modern carotid stenting techniques were available.) I had already performed over 800 carotid endarterectomies (surgical procedures to remove atherosclerotic plaque) with outstanding results. I also had the only accredited non-invasive vascular laboratory in the surrounding three counties that could perform diagnostic vascular studies (with a high degree of consistent accuracy). I have included a complete description of this procedure in the Appendix B.

I agreed entirely with the consultants that he needed to undergo this procedure. I met with him, his wife, and one of his daughters to consider and review the procedure. As we prepared him for surgery, I knew that he trusted me and understood the risks involved (including stroke).

The procedure was as flawless as any we'd ever done. However, once the patient woke up from the anesthesia, we were shocked to find that he was paralyzed on the right side and was unable to speak. To say that I was devastated was an understatement.

Immediately, we reopened the blood vessel to ensure it had not thrombosed. We found that this was not the case. We then performed an arteriogram to identify anything that might have caused this complication, but nothing emerged. We concluded that some tiny bit of plaque may have broken off, perhaps when we positioned his head and turned him sideways before even making the incision. He was in the intensive care unit for an entire week. He did not die, but he made very little progress. His wound healed, and the stitches were removed, but he needed to be transferred to rehabilitation. We all hoped that he would make some improvement. However, as the days went by, it was clear that this was not happening. His wife and daughter told me they did not blame me and knew I had done my best. Eventually, they returned home.

A few months later I was at a meeting of the American Venous Forum. I was still upset over the outcome of this procedure, and even though my stroke rate was only 0.8% (well below the national average of 2 to 3%), I was debating with myself as to whether I should stop doing carotid surgery. I was simply overwhelmed, and I felt that maybe I needed to stop. In other words, perhaps it's me!

Dr Norman Rich, one of the giants in American Vascular Surgery, Past President of The Society for Vascular Surgery, and who was then the Chief of Surgery at Walter Reed National Military Medical Center (now known as National Naval Medical Center), was among the faculty present at this meeting. I did not know him at all other than to say "hello, Sir," and he certainly did not know me. Nonetheless, I summoned my courage, approached him during the reception, and said, *"Doctor Rich, can I talk to you for a second? I want to talk to you as if I was a parishioner and you were the Priest."* He must have thought I was out of my mind, and I went on to tell him how demoralized I was and that I thought I should stop doing carotid surgery. He thought for a moment and then asked me what the indications were, how I did the procedure, what my training was, and how many procedures I'd done.

He said, *"Listen, you've got a long career ahead of you, and you're as good as they come in the community and as good as they come anywhere, so you go back there and get back on the diving board. It doesn't mean you don't feel bad, but it's happened to me and may happen to you again."* So, I decided to continue as a carotid surgeon.

Many months later, I received a personal letter in my office with a return address I didn't recognize. This letter was from another of my patient's daughters, one who had not been here in Florida during her father's surgery.

A Letter from My Patient's Daughter

Doctor Lynn,

I just want to say that I have never met you but you took away something very precious to me.

On February 20, 2004 my father Ted C. entrusted his life to you but you performed a botched surgery and took away most of his world as he knew it. He was very excited about this surgery because he so feared having a stroke. After your surgery he never walked or was able to tell his kids that he loved them again.

He suffered for 10 months. We brought him home to Indiana and my mother took care of his every need. My mom and my sisters and I had to do tasks for him that took away every bit of dignity he had left. Because even though he couldn't move you could tell by his eyes that he still knew what was going on. On December 11 his suffering ended. He passed away.

Only you know what happened that day but something went terribly wrong. Maybe it is time for you to retire and enjoy your family the way my Dad will not be able to.

Sincerely,
Your Patient's Daughter

This was quite a blow. I was hurt and deeply saddened, especially after Dr Rich kindly guided me through this. Although I felt beaten up and demoralized, I still believed that I needed to try to explain and help her understand exactly what had happened. I sent her the following letter dated January 22, 2005.

℘ A Letter to My Patient's Daughter

Dear Ms. D.,

I received your letter and, needless to say, was deeply troubled by the content. First and foremost, I am very sorry that your father, Ted C., has passed away and I can assure you, despite never having met you, that your mother and your sister knew that I did everything possible during the operation, immediately after the operation and daily in my devotion to your father's care. I can understand your sense of loss and I am quite lucky to still have both my mother and father at 85 years of age who are with me. I dread the day that they are gone.

As I hope you know, your father was operated upon because of a critical carotid lesion and having had a previous stroke. The situation was of urgency and I can tell you that I have the reputation, and have continued to maintain it, that every possible attention to detail is always covered. This includes before the surgery, intraoperatively and obviously during the surgery and postoperatively. There was no question but that your father needed the procedure. I can tell you that, having performed over 800 carotid endarterectomies diligently; I have had a total of four strokes, your father having been the last. That is well below the national average in the best centers in the world but it is not at zero. For someone such as your father's situation, the risk of stroke was anywhere between 1 and 5-6 percent in anyone's hands at any university. It is unfortunately inherent in the basic process and, despite perfect technique and despite all attention to detail with magnifying loops, head lamps, two vascular surgeons at the operating table and an experienced team with anesthesia, these rare but devastating events may sometimes occur. Obviously they can occur even before the operation, such as what happened with your father.

If I had his operation to do over again, I can honestly tell you that, critically looking at it, things would be done the same way. Strokes occur whether the patient is done under general anesthesia or whether the patient is done awake under cervical block, whether one uses a patch or does not use a patch, etc.

Approximately one month after your father's event, I was at the American Venous Forum, a prestigious vascular society and spoke to Doctor Norman Rich, who is one of the giants in vascular surgery and who was head of Walter Reed for many, many years and a pioneer in carotid surgery. I spoke to him as a parishioner would speak to a priest telling him how badly I felt and how demoralized, if you will, I was after your father's stroke. He reassured me when he realized the way the procedure had been carried out and the number of procedures I have performed and counseled me as to the fact that this is unfortunately the nature of the specialty and the nature of the procedure. It is no different than a plane crash. If one flies on an airline and wants a guarantee that the plane will not crash, there is no airline in the world that will sell the passenger the ticket, yet we all take the plane and hope for the best and thank G-d we are all still here, but not everyone is and we have all read about the unfortunate totally gentle, non-harmful people who perish for no explainable reason.

I know from my conversations with your sister, Sherry R., that she understood my compassion and my dedication to your father. I would recommend that you read a book entitled "*Doctors Cry, Too, Essays from the Heart of a Physician*" by Frank H. Boehm, M.D. It is a book that I have read and, infact, I have met Doctor Boehm and it shows in a unique way that doctors are subject to the same stresses and pressures in life as everyone else and that physicians suffer equally as much as patients' families.

There is never a night that goes by that when the phone rings at 2:00, 3:00, or 4:00 in the A.M. from the ICU that all of the potential possibilities of problems go through my mind and immediately I deal with it. I was very fond of your father and mother and felt privileged that they came all the way from Okeechobee to be cared for by me. I can only tell you that I did my best and I believe that is all that one can do. I am deeply sorry for your feelings and I am confident that, had you been at the hospital and met me, perhaps your feelings would have been different from the standpoint of compassion, caring and reputation heard from the professionals within the hospital with whom I work. I am not in any way trying to brag or boast but to try in some way to let you know that I too have a heart and a conscience and I am committed every single time that I am given the privilege of caring for someone to carry out a procedure to the best of my ability. I was trained at Harvard by a perfectionist whose picture is staring at me at this moment in my office as I dictate this letter and he never, ever took an operation, no matter how complex or minor in a light way. He had a famous saying that "there is no such thing as minor surgery, only minor surgeons." Obviously carotid endarterectomy was not minor and is not minor but, on the other hand, just because one has done 800 procedures, each one has to be as if it was your first with the same attention to detail and I can assure you that this was the case with your father on that day.

I hope that you will feel some degree of comfort from this letter and I hope that you share it with your mother and your sister. I am available to you at any time should you need to speak to me for further closure and I wish you peace and continued fond memories of your father. As I stated at the beginning I am lucky at this moment in time that I still have my father and for that I am deeply sorry for you but your father is at peace and, in my conscience, I am hopeful that he looks favorably upon me.

With deep respect and sorrow for your loss,
I remain,
Richard A. Lynn, M.D., F.A.C.S.

Although some of my colleagues thought otherwise, I was not doing this to prevent a lawsuit. Most of my colleagues and some of my dearest friends told me that I should not have done this. They said, "Let it go; if you get sued, you get sued." Looking back at this now, 15 or more years later, I remain convinced I did not write this letter to attempt to block a lawsuit. Maybe I needed to provide myself with some closure.

Three years later, in March 2008, I received another letter from my patient's daughter.

☙ A Response from My Patient's Daughter

Dear Dr. Lynn,

First, I must say I apologize that I am just now sending you this letter. I should have sent it three years ago but I was grieving over the loss of my father and needed someone to blame and unfortunately you were the one that I chose.

I am not sure you remember me or not but my father, Ted C., had a stroke and died 10 months later after you performed carotid artery surgery on him. I then wrote you a seething letter blaming you for my loss. I knew better to than blame you, and my Dad would have been very disappointed in me for doing so but unfortunately I did it anyway.

I was going through some items in my desk today and found the letter you sent to me in response to my letter. I really appreciate the time you took out of your busy life to send it to me. When I received your letter it made me realize what a compassionate man you are and also that doctors also hurt when something happens to their patients. I was also pleased that you remembered my Dad and that he wasn't just a number but that you were also devastated by what happened to him.

My Dad really looked up to you and I should have known that he would not have entrusted his life to someone who was not a kind and caring person as well as talented in his field. So when I found the letter that you sent me, I also felt a nudge by a wonderful angel that I needed to help you too find some peace in all of this.

So, Dr. Lynn, please accept my apology for the letter I sent to you. I was Daddy's girl and was totally devastated by losing him. I just want you to know that I wish you nothing but peace and happiness in your life.

Sincerely,
Your Patient's Daughter

You can imagine how I felt when I got this. I cried, literally cried in my office. Here I was, just going through my mail, and I had a busy office day ahead of me. Nonetheless, I somehow got ahold of her telephone number, and I called her. When she answered the phone, I said, *"This is Dr Lynn; please don't hang up."* At the time, I didn't know if she really meant what she said. To make a long story short, we spoke for an entire hour, and she told me that she had been going through many difficult situations at that time and felt guilty about not being there for her father. I thanked her from the bottom of my heart and told her about my family, my kids, and my grandchildren. She went on to tell me about her mom.

I saved this correspondence; maybe I knew then that I would have the opportunity to share this with you now, so many years later.

When all was said and done, the most important part was that I felt that she genuinely forgave me. We all must recognize that our patients and their families are only human. I was glad that I sent the letter, as long and verbose as it was. Honestly, I looked up from my desk, and Dr Silen's picture was staring at me. I know that I did what he would have wanted me to do.

Remember, this is not about a carotid endarterectomy, the practice of surgery, or me. This is about the lifelong commitment that you are about to undertake.

Before moving on, I refer you back to the quote from the Mayo brothers, who remarked on the tremendous responsibility of having a patient's life in your hands. Keep sight of this important fact, no matter your chosen specialty. We all understand how hard this can be when, for example, you are tired and busy and faced with a patient here for another repeat emergency visit with the same complaint. It isn't easy to remain idealistic and focused 24 hours a day and seven days a week, but you must try.

Also, remember to seek out mentors. You need at least one or two mentors who will lead the way, guide you, and provide you with a path forward, even if just metaphorically, and even when you are forty years into your career.

CHAPTER EIGHT

Articles of Interest

THE FOLLOWING ARTICLES may interest you as you embark on your careers. A complete reference list, including all the information needed to locate each of these publications online, can be found at the end of this chapter.

℘ 1. The Qualities of a Good Surgeon by Ephraim McDowell

This article briefly describes the life and times of Ephraim McDowell, an eminent American surgeon who practiced in Kentucky in the late 1700s and early 1800s.

This artcile highlights the essential traits and skills needed for surgical excellence. McDowell emphasizes that a good surgeon must possess technical expertise, steady hands, and a deep understanding of anatomy. Equally important are personal qualities like compassion, patience, and the ability to remain calm under pressure.

He also stresses the importance of lifelong learning and staying up-to-date with medical advancements. A good surgeon must build patient trust, demonstrating empathy and clear communication. McDowell concludes that a successful surgeon blends medical skills with strong ethical principles, always prioritizing the well-being of their patients.

2. Surgical Education: In need of a paradigm shift by Dr William Silen

In a 2003 article in the *New England Journal of Medicine*, my mentor, Dr William Silen, shared his deep concerns about changes in surgical training programs. Although retired from practice by then, he observed that current students and trainees were not often given a chance to learn directly from preeminent physicians at the bedside—witnessing skills like abdominal palpation or listening for heart murmurs and carotid bruits. Instead, training increasingly relied on scans and imaging. Dr Silen firmly believed that programs needed to return to these essential, hands-on basics. Sadly, this shift back has not materialized. Given modern demands like finances, relative value units, and the pace of today's surgical practice, I think he sensed it might never happen. He knew that few surgeons would still be willing to arrive at the hospital at 5:00 AM to teach, as he had in earlier years.

꧂ 3. Mourning on Morning Rounds by Mounsica Vallurupalli, B.S.

Mourning on Morning Rounds, by Mounsica Vallurupalli, B.S., offers a deeply personal account of the emotional challenges faced by medical professionals. Written by a medical student, the article reflects on her feelings after the loss of a patient who suffered cardiac arrest and died in the intensive care unit. Vallurupalli explores the tension between maintaining professionalism and experiencing genuine grief, emphasizing the need to balance compassion with resilience. Her insights highlight the profound and universal nature of these emotions, helping readers better understand the human side of medicine.

꧂ 4. From Illness as Culture to Caregiving as a Moral Experience by Dr Arthur Kleinman

From Illness as Culture to Caregiving as a Moral Experience, by Dr Arthur Kleinman, published in 2008 in the *Journal of the American Medical Association*'s "A Piece of My Mind" section, offers a personal and cultural reflection on illness and caregiving. As a physician and the primary caregiver for his wife after her Alzheimer's diagnosis, Kleinman shares how this experience deepened his empathy for others in similar situations. He explores caregiving as a moral and human experience, emphasizing the importance of understanding what life is like "on the other side of the fence." The article calls for greater recognition of the emotional and ethical challenges caregivers face.

☙ 5. Listening to Leviticus by Mark Twain

Listening to Leviticus, by Mark Twain, referenced by a surgeon, reflects on the complexities of interpreting religious texts and their impact on modern decisions. The piece discusses a surgeon's experience with a Jehovah's Witness patient, whose faith prohibits blood transfusions based on Leviticus 3:17. Twain's satirical critique of literal scriptural interpretation is juxtaposed with the surgeon's real-life challenge of respecting a patient's deeply held beliefs while providing care. This article offers valuable insights into viewing patients holistically and understanding how to approach medical procedures with empathy and respect for their cultural and religious values.

☙ 6. Oliver Wendell Holmes and the "Dimple" Artifact by Dr Andrew L. Warshaw

The final article in this collection was written by Dr Andrew Warshaw and published in 2013 in the journal *Surgery*. Dr Warshaw was the Chair of the Department of Surgery at Massachusetts General Hospital at Harvard

Medical School for 20 years and then went on to become the President of the American College of Surgeons.

The article explores the historical and medical significance of a unique anatomical observation made by Oliver Wendell Holmes, a prominent physician and writer. Dr Warshaw delves into Holmes's keen powers of observation, highlighting how this seemingly minor detail—referred to as the "dimple" artifact—reflected Holmes's contributions to understanding human anatomy and clinical practice. The article celebrates Holmes's legacy as a physician who bridged science and the humanities. I played a prominent role in this story! I hope that you will read it in its entirety.

☙ REFERENCES ❧

1. Othersen HB Jr. Ephraim McDowell: the qualities of a good surgeon. *Ann Surg*. 2004;239(5):648-650. doi:10.1097/01.sla.0000124382.04128.5a

2. Silen W. Surgical education: in need of a shift in paradigm. *Surgery*. 2003;134(2):399-402. doi:10.1067/msy.2003.232

3. Vallurupalli M. Mourning on morning rounds. *N Engl J Med*. 2013;369(5):404-405. doi:10.1056/NEJMp1300969

4. Kleinman A. From illness as culture to caregiving as moral experience. *N Engl J Med*. 2013;368(15):1376-1377. doi:10.1056/NEJMp1300678

5. Campbell BH. A piece of my mind. Listening to leviticus. *JAMA*. 2008;299(8):879-880. doi:10.1001/jama.299.8.879

6. Warshaw AL. Oliver Wendell Holmes and the "dimple" artifact. *Surgery*. 2013;153(2):292-293. doi:10.1016/j.surg.2011.07.042

Conclusion

As you turn the final pages of this book, I hope it has touched your heart, sparked meaningful reflections, or even guided you toward pivotal decisions. If this work has inspired you to consider what it truly means to be a physician or surgeon, or if it has awakened in you a desire to do more, learn more, or be more, it has achieved its purpose.

Medicine and surgery are not just professions—they are profound callings that demand compassion, resilience, and an unyielding commitment to humanity. We can make a difference, not only with our hands but with our hearts and minds. As you progress in your journey, remember that the most extraordinary impact often comes from the simplest acts of care and understanding.

If you have questions, ideas, or personal stories to share—or if this book has resonated with you in any way—I would be honored to connect with you. Please feel free to reach out to me via email or phone. Your thoughts and experiences are invaluable, and I would welcome the opportunity to engage in a meaningful dialogue.

Let this be my final charge to you: embrace your role as a healer with humility and courage, hold steadfast to the values that define this sacred profession, and always strive to make the world a little brighter for those you serve. Together, we can uphold the timeless principles of medicine and inspire future generations to carry them forward.

Thank you for allowing me to share my story with you. Now, create your own story. One filled with purpose, passion, and unwavering integrity.

Richard A. Lynn, MD, FACS, RPVI
rich549bux@gmail.com
+1 (561) 315-6208

Appendix A

This is the original Survival Manual distributed to incoming interns at the Beth Israel/Harvard Department of Surgery. It was created by a former resident who, after repeatedly failing to follow Dr. Silen's directives, was tasked with writing a guide to ensure future trainees would have no excuse for "not listening."

HOUSE OFFICIERS' SURVIVAL MANUAL

"YOU GUYS NEVER LISTEN" - A REBUTTAL

DEDICATION

To Dr. Silen, a great surgeon and teacher,

without whom there would be no need for this manual.

The following collection of random ideas has been gathered without effort at any specific organization. An attempt to assist the house officier searching for information on a specific subject has been made by entitling each entry with the main subject of that entry.

BANDAGES AND DRESSINGS

DO NOT TOUCH ANY DRESSING WITHOUT DR. SILEN'S EXPRESSION PERMISSION AND KNOWLEDGE OF SUCH.

As there is no bleeding intraoperatively, it is not necessary to use a large bulky postop dressing. Several layers of 4x4's are adequate. The skin surrounding the wound is painted with benzoin (don't use the spray benzoin) and after it gets tacky the wound may be dressed with either adhesive tape if you;re in the OR or paper tape if you're on the floor.

In biliary surgery, drain sites are dressed separately such that the dressing over the drain can be lifted up and the drain slipped out at the 24-36th hour post-op (if it is not draining bile).

CHOLANGIOGRAMS

A. Diagnostic cholangiograms - as stated later under xray preps, there is no such thing as a routine prep. Specifically, there is no prep usually ordered for the T-tube cholangiogram and the so-called "routine" prep prescribed by the xray dept. is an atom bomb compared with the gentle prep of MOM that Dr. Silen's usually prefers.

B. OR cholangiogram -

a. The requisition - be sure to fill this out before coming to the OR - at least before the operation commences. Forge-ting to do this kills much time in the OR, much running around, and alot of gastric secretion on both the part of Dr. Silen and his resident.

b. Positioning of patients for intra-operative cholangiograms -

1. Check to see that the grid is on the OR table - before the patient is on same.
2. Draw an imaginary line starting at the right mid-clavicular point until it crosses the right costal margin. At its intersection with the right costal margin draw a 2nd line perpendicular to the 1st - this second line should be the mid-point of the xray plate (most xray grids have an eye-screw with a string or adhesive tape marker on their sides to mark this mid-point.)
3. The patient must be over to the right so that he is almost flush with the side of the gird.

DRAINS

Drains do not stop bleeding. Drains are to be used only for specific purposes - as in biliary tract surgery, to drain bile.

Drains should not drain blood.

Drains are bug chutes.

THE EIGHT O'CLOCK CALL

After 8 p.m. when the 8 o'clock temps are supposed to be taken but never are make rounds to collect these temps (usually this means requesting that they be taken on Dr. Silen's patients) and make quicky rounds on the patients.

A call at 9 p.m. will be made to Dr. Silen to report this information; be prepared to bring him up-to-date on important I & O's.

Do hct's on those patients whose fluid balance is tenuous or rapidly changing.

HISTORY

"If you listen, the patient will tell you what's the matter with him."

I & O

Every patient on IV's and beginning oral alimentation should have an I&O summary sheet filled out by the HO himself.

Weight should be recorded daily - when pertinent, hcts, lytes, etc. should also be noted on the sheet.

Keep the sheet up-to-date - besides the fact that Dr. Silen insists on it, you can't write for fluids accurately without the info it collects for you.

Don't leave the filling out of this sheet until the last minute before rounds in the morning because invariably there is one I&O - always on your sickest patient, the one with the most tubes plus an ileostomy - which requires some deciferring. In general, it is best to get this task done as soon after 12MN as possible, so that the appropriate nightingale can be called and asked to explain her contribution to the confusion.

Keep a running total of the mEq. of Na and K given in the course of the day - there are spaces for this on the sheet under Intake.

A word of advice: when the 3 holes on the sheet wear out and the sheet is found floating free in the chart, attach gummed reenforcements before it gets lost (it will for sure - then you're stuck with the choice of catching hell for letting it get lost or the monumentous task of redoing the sheet from the old I&O's.

INSTRUMENTS

1. Dressing forceps - in the OR, do not use them. Use instead a long straight clamp. With dressing forceps you are unable to clamp any bleeders; they are bulky; they slow you up.
2. The clamp - the clamp referred to above is not to be used to poke - sooner or later you'll poke a hole through the bowel.
3. Kelly clamps - "All good surgical house officiers have Kelly clamps."
   A. In the OR, a Kelly is not a Kelly, it is a Mayo.
4. Scissors - "All good surgical house officiers have bandage scissors."

MEDEX

The medex is to be checked each and every morning before rounds for every patient noting the type and frequency of medications.

Note particularly the frequency of pain meds and also the time of day it is given -if it is being given the same time every day, this suggest that it is the nursing staff passing out meds rather than the patient requesting

Check especially that all important meds such as antibiotics have been give

Pain and sleep meds should be written on a day to day basis - no standing orders permitted initially in the patient's hospital course - this is subject to change later.

Meds which have a changing dosage schedule such as steroids should be written for on a daily basis writing for the dose for the following day the preceding morning, thus Tuesday's dose is written for on Monday morning.

IN THE OR

1. Arteries - large arteries (and ducts) are ligated with 00 silk plus a 000 silk suture ligature.

B. Drapes
1. The drape itself - drapes are used as they come from the sterile pack - folded in half - folding and refolding drapes is a waste of time and lends itself to contamination.
2. Draping - drapes folded in half as they are straight out of the pack are placed on the operative field - on cases in which xrays may be taken, they are sewn in place using a heavy cutting needle. In tying these drapes down, the resident is reportedly contaminated invariably by himself.
While draping the betadine sterile prep is left alone.
Dr. Silen does not use sticky drapes and does not go through the rigamarol of blotting off the betadine.
3. Skin drapes - Dr. Silen uses two skin drapes around the abdominal wound and these are either sewn in or clamped with towel clips to the skin.
a. Technique - Hold a toothed forceps in one hand and grasp the edge of the skin; feed the towel to the skin edge so that it may then be fix in place.

C. Hemostasis - when vessel are clamped, the hold the clamp as it is placed on the vessel - don't twist the clamp around.

D. The appropriate hesitation - it is appropriate, indeed, mandatory that one hesitate after pulling a needle thru tissue - this enables Dr. Silen to grasp the tail of the suture that is within the eye of the needle and begin tying his knot smoothly.
a. It is also mandatory that one hesitate before removing a clamp on a vessel - this is necessary so that you are sure he has placed his knot securely.

E. The incision - as Dr. Silen makes his incision one should have in his left hand a sponge to provide traction and in his right hand a snap - a straight snap - always keep a straight snap or some instrument in your right hand.
a. As the incision is made gentle traction is placed on the skin.
b. Be sure not to place too much traction on the skin or he will accuse you of skewing the wound.
c. In the are of the xiphoid, extending the skin incision for an inch above the tip of the xiphoid is a key manuever - "in this are, an inch is worth a mile."

F. Packing off the wound - In packing off a wound, as in all other aspects of life, position is everything.
a. Do not use too many packs and do not wad the pack into the wound.

G. Prep table - sterile towels should be placed around the edges of the prep table and while the anesthetist is messing around, the prep table is brought over to the operating table and the resident stands posed to begin his scrub as soon as the intubation is complete.

H. Surgical scrub - 2 sterile towels should be placed on either side of the patient running from the axilla along the mid-axillary line down as far they will go.
a. 10 minute prep - a GENTLE 10 minute by the clock surgical scrub with betadine should be performed by the resident. The resident need not have scrubbed himself first before doing the surgical prep. If he has not scrubbed yet, he merely wears a pair of sterile gloves and scrubs himself afterwards while Dr. Silen is draping the patient. If he has already scrubbed, he should then gown and glove and do the 10 minute prep and then change gown and gloves.
1. After the 10 minute prep, 2 dry towels are used to blot the moisted skin.

2. One cannot over-emphasize the gentleness of this prep because too vigorous scrubbing of the skin causes hyperemia and excessive bleeding - "I'll lose more blood on the skin incision than the rest of the operation."

I. Sponging - when sponging the wound, do not wipe but tamp the area.

J. Sterile technique - breech of sterile technique drives him bananas.

a. From the resident's point of view, keep in mind the following - only the "strike zone" is an area of sterility; that is, from the top of the shoulders to the waist waist

b. Do not fold the arms and place gloved hands in the axillae.

c. It is acceptable to place the hands in the pouches of the gowns, but these gowns are being phased out with the purchase of new ones - which do not have pouches - there is the risk that the cloth hidden from view may be defective.

K. Suction - Put a Mayo (Kelley) clamp on the suction tubing so that it does not hiss throughout the case when it is not needed.

L. What to do - "Don't just stand there, do something!"

ORDERS

A. Orders are to be written so that they are idiot-proof.

B. Orders should be written well beneath the preceding orders so that no new orders are missed.

C. Orders should be numbered and a line skipped between each new numbered order.

D. Orders which are important or out of the ordinary should be brought to the attention of the head nurse and the nurse who will be carrying out that order.

E. Pre-op orders should include an order to have the patient void at 5a.m. and weighed in at that time on the morning of the operation.

a. Note: you should plan to put in all IVs, CVPs, Foleys, NG tubes, etc. at this time too.

F. Anesthesia pre-op orders need to be checked carefully - they sometimes get carried away with their doseages of pre-meds compounding the post-op problems created by their intra-operative poisons.

G. Pre-op orders are to be written so that they can be checked by Dr. Silen on rounds the morning prior to the day of surgery (but not too soon, or the nightingales will screw it up - not earlier than midnight the night before the morning prior to the day of the surgery).

PRE-OP PREPARATION

A. Re: the johnny and the IV - a pet peeve of the Dr. Silen's is to have the IV inserted with the patient's arm still within the sleeve of the johnny on the morning of the operation - thus, the patient arrives in the OR and a lot of dancing around ensues while extracating the patient and his IV bottles and lines from the clutches of the johnny

B. The prep - check to see that the patient has been prepped before he leaves his room.

a. On all abdominal cases, include nipples to groin.

POST-OP CARE

A. Oxygen - almost every patient with an upper abdominal incision is to have face mask O_2 for 24 hours post-op.

B. Voiding - it is the resident's responsibility to see and encourage and stimulate the patient to void post-operatively - he must visit the patient every 30-45 minutes until he has voided or until you and Dr. Silen are convinced that it is a lost cause and a Foley is called for.

a. God help the resident who has to cath a "neglected" patient.

b. Check that the patient is not distended and does not have the desire to void on supra-pubic compression.

c. Dr. Silen will be irritated with you even if you are with him himself doing something that is necessary and appropriate whenn he realizes that a post-op patient hasn't been attending to.

1. It is better to excuse yourself and the check the patient - rarely he will absolve you of this responsibility.

PROGRESS NOTES

A. Each progress note is to be headed by the date, time, and post-op day number.

B. If available the 8p.m. temp should be included in the heading.

C. The following categories are suggested:

a. Sx - include how the patient feels and other subjective items

b. P.E. - lungs, all sites of current and past IVs, plus the area of the pathology

c. Lab data - heme, bacti, chem, xray, EKG

d. Impression - how you put it all together with the pros and cons

e. Plans

f. Signature - if a medical student has written this note it is necessary to read it and countersign it prior to morning rounds

D. Notes in the chart reflect one's thimking.

PACKING

Dr. Silen dislikes (abhors) the "pernicious practice of post-operative packing."

ROUNDS

A. Morning rounds should be made prior to Dr. Silen's arrival at 6a.m. Mondays thru Saturdays and at 9a/m/ on Sundays and holidays.

a. It is suggested that you begin no later than 5a.m. on non-operating days and no later than 4a.m. on operating days until you get the hang of it.

B. A Check-list is helpful with the following items to be accomplished for each patient: 1. check the I&O summary sheet, 2. make sure a 5a.m. weight is available for round, 3. write all orders, 4. check the medex, 5. countersign all student notes, 6. do P.E. on each patient

a. Additional task may be necessary in special instances like irrigating a tube, changing a dressing as in an AP resection, etc.

C. Re: the P.E. - don't forget to scrutinize the patient for phebitis = Dr. Silen is a bug on this - it is also a great cop-out for an unexplaine fever

D. Re: I&O - have an approximate idea the I&O from MN to the beginning of rounds

E. Keep a list of all lab data ordered - Dr. Silen will ask what they are on evening rounds even tho the lab sheets aren't back yet from the labs

a. This necessitates calling the lab during the day after the desired test has been run

b. It is easiest when students are on the service to assign each student a patient and make that patient and everything about him that student' responsibility - this way you have some one person to ask what and why not - he should get the lab data he orders on his patient and whatever he doesn't do by a reasonable time, just do yourself - this approach saves a lot of hell on the resident and gives the student his crack at carrying the ball - if he blows then you have to step in to save yourself (and the patient) by a dressing cart you can pick up a debridement set, gloves, 4x4's, betadine, steri-strips, benzoin, etc., etc. on the way to the patient's room - this saves a lot of leg work.

G. Try to see all xrays before Dr. Silen does - he loves to pick up things that HOs and radiologists miss.

THE SERMONS

A. The pre-op sermon - the sermon is a speech given to each patient pre-operatively - it is designed to explained what the respiratory problem is post-op and how best to avoid problems. There is also a small demonstration showing the patient how the respiratory effort is increased after abdominal incisions and showing him how to exercise his legs.

a. The Sermon:

1. Why the problem - secretions collect in the lungs and plug bronchial tubes which leads to atelectasis and pneumonia.
2. How to avoid the problem - take 10 deep breathes and cough x 3 every hour to raise phlegm. Remind the patient that nonproductive coughing is still important and shows what a good job he is doing in clearing his secretions.
3. Will my stitches break? - every patient worries about this post-operatively and this is something which should not worry the patient. Assure him that he will not bust open, even with the most vigorous coughing.
4. Post-op discomfort (N.B.: avoid using the word pain) - medicine will be available for incisional discomfort which may occur during deep breathing and coughing - this discomfort is not harmful -the medicine will take the edge off the discomfort - but don't expect it to abolish the discomfort.
5. Demonstration - have the patient take a deep breathe lying relaxed in bed. Then have him lift his head off the pillow and take a deep breathe. Comment that this restriction in respiratory effort is very similar to that experienced post-operatively.
6. Leg exercises - dorsiflex the feet and wiggle the legs 30 or so times an hour.

B. The discharge sermon - specific instructions may vary with varying procedures but in general the following are applicable to all abdominal cases:

a. Do what you feel what to doing including driving (mention that driving should be put off until the patient feels that fear of incisional disfomfort is pretty much gone - being afraid to turn around to see what's coming because of pain is a relative contraindication to driving)
b. Do not lift anything heavier than your (wife's) pocketbook for 6 weeks
c. Anticipate that you will get tired easily.
d. Don't bathe until at least 12-14 days post-op, and/or until the sutures have been removed (including retentions).

SUTURES

A. Skin suture - placing of

a. Skin sutures should be placed one cm. apart and one cm. in width.
b. They should be alternating - simple and mattress sutures.
c. There should be no tension with a skin suture.

B. Suture removal

a. When removing sutures as well as stays, the wound is first painted with betadine, sterilely of course.
b. The sutures are then individually cut, each away from the knot.

c. The para-wound area is painted with benzoin.
d. Then with steri-strips ready, the sutures are removed one at a time and steri-strips are applied as you go.

C. As long as there are any sutures in the the wound, a dressing is employed.

TUBOLOGY

A. Tubology is the art and science of handling tubes, specifically in this context, the NG tube.

B. Type of tube - for nasogastric intubation, a #14 Levine tube is used
a. For decompression in the usual situations, this tube is adequate and as comfortable as you can get - larger tubes for routine use are unnecessarily uncomfortable.
b. In the bleeding patient or patient with food in the stomach, even an #18 is too small to empty the stomach - an Ewald tube is then used.

C. Passing the tube - in general, a tube is passed while allowing the patient to have sips of water.

D. Taping the tube to patient - use ½" tape (adhesive), long enough to run from the forehead, down the nose, and onto the tube for a couple of inches.
a. At the point where the tape begins to run over the tube, split the tape in two and wrap the tails around the tube in opposite directions.

E. Connection the tube up - the tube is usually connected to a Gomco suction machine. The following points are worthy of note as they drive him nuts when he sees they are overlooked.
a. Check that the glass rubber junction where the tube fits over the glass connector is not a spot for kinking of the tube - be sure that the tube is well seated on the glass connector to avoid this.
b. Check to see that the machine itself is a working number - there are several units which never work and never get fixed.

F. Positioning the tube - position is everything in life and this is true in tubology also.
a. Starting at the anterior nares, roughly two black lines should be visible. This has proved to be an excellent guideline.

G. Irrigating the tube - unnecessary!!
a. Irrigation is necessary only when there is food or clot in the stomach - see above.

H. Malfunctioning tubes - check to see that you are hooked up to a working Gomco and that there is no kinking in the lines esp. at the glass-rubbe junction.

XRAYS

A. Seeing them - look at <u>all</u> available xrays on every patient
a. You'll be amased what others have missed.

B. Prepping for them - nothing is routine - remember this and you make out alright.

GLOTZERY OF TERMS, QUOTES, AND MISC.

Silen's First Law: "Doctors are dangerous."

Rosoff's Corollary: "Some more so than others."

Surgery: "Surgery is all detail."

The Scrub Nurse: "the chastity belt of the OR."

Flea: Mope: Swarmi: medical man or internist.

Flea Circus: Medical service.

Fat Boy: basically term of endearment - - note tone though.

Big Boy: same as Fat Boy.

Halstead

Red cell: that which should not be seen in the OR.

ERBCL = Estimated Red Blood Cell Loss: Silen's version of the EBL.

Nuggerin': a descriptive term of an action or motion which Dr. Silen interprets as indecisive, inept, inappropriate, unecessary, dangerous, wasteful, repetitious, mistimed, miscalculated, unadvisable, stupid

Sitting on it: "Stay on it, sit on it, don't play with it."

"I feel a memorandum coming on."

"There are no mysteries in medicine, just mysterious doctors."

"Do it in your spare time."

"Make the anastomosis in heaven and the patient goes to hell."

"Pull up a loose stool."

"Come into my orifice."

"If I could only be my own first assistant."

"The New England Journal of, excuse the expression, Medicine."

"Hell, he lost less blood during that operation than he would if he underwent a medical work-up."

"Iatrogenesis imperfecta profunda."

"Get the light somewhere in the vicinity of Massachusetts."

"Just like night follows day."

"B.S." = before Silen.

"Better to be lucky than smart."

"Get that damn fleatern down here and show him what a real gallbladder looks like."

"If you're a good boy..."

"You guys never listen!" - IF YOU STILL BELIEVE THAT, DR. SILEN, SEE THE ABOVE!

Appendix B

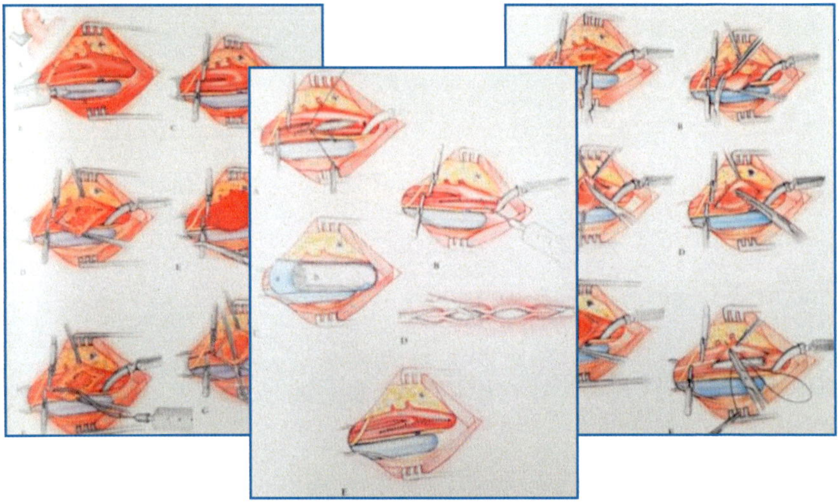

In years past, carotid endarterectomy was the only procedure available to treat atherosclerotic disease of the carotid arteries. To begin, imagine the patient's head is turned to the side, and an incision is made along the sternocleidomastoid muscle. The carotid artery and jugular vein can be found at a site a few layers beneath this muscle. The internal carotid artery extends up to the brain, and the external carotid provides blood to the face.

Atherosclerotic debris can break loose from carotid plaques and form emboli that can move up to the brain, resulting in stroke. Sometimes, these are small strokes called transient ischemic attacks (TIAs). A TIA can be caused by a tiny piece of plaque that breaks off and lodges in the patient's brain for a few minutes to a few hours (but fewer than 24 hours), which can lead to *transient* blindness or weakness on one side and/or an inability to speak. Not all patients experience TIAs. In some cases, the very first ischemic episode can be devastating, debilitating, and potentially life-threatening.

Then, the carotid artery is prepared for clamping. Next, the patient will receive appropriate anticoagulant medication to prevent clotting. However, no blood is going to the brain on this side, although you can consider placing a shunt if necessary. The artery is opened, and the atherosclerotic plaque is removed. The artery is then closed with or without a patch. Additional details on this procedure can be found in most vascular surgery textbooks.

The purpose of the preceding paragraphs was not to go into great detail on the procedure itself but to highlight its overall intricacy. For many years, this was always my favorite procedure. But eventually, I began to hate it. How did this happen? Put simply, even if the operation was technically perfect, once you closed the skin, you had to sit with your "fingers crossed" until the patient woke from general anesthesia (95% of the cases were done in this way) to make sure that the patient could move everything, and articulate appropriately. One of the significant risks of this procedure was an intraoperative stroke. Through no fault of your own, a small piece of plaque could break loose during the procedure, and upon awakening, the patient could be paralyzed on one side. In the best and most experienced hands, the incidence of an intraoperative stroke is roughly 2 to 4 percent and somewhat higher in symptomatic high-risk patients. After 25 years of performing this procedure under general anesthesia, a respected anesthesiologist colleague of mine suggested that I might try this procedure on a patient who remained awake under local anesthesia. While I was very anxious about drastically changing my protocol, I trusted him and his expertise, and I eventually gave this a try.

I saw that there were several advantages to this approach. The left carotid artery supplies blood to the left side of the brain, and the left side of the brain controls the right side of the body. You can communicate with the patient throughout the procedure if he remains awake. You can put a squeaky ball in his right hand and ask him to keep squeezing it; if he can follow your directions, you know that he's mentating appropriately, and there's no need to put in a shunt. After trying this once, I never returned to the old way of doing things.

*Reflections from the Audience**

"Just as you have, I will work to remember my roots and give back to the communities who need it most. I was blown away by the story you gave about the patient who underwent a stroke during a carotid endarterectomy. As you said, life is 10% what happens to you and 90% how you deal with it. How you dealt with his daughter shows your true moral character as an astounding and empathic human being and that you are someone others should try to emulate. I will try my best to show the same professionalism and class that you portrayed, and I hope one day to embody the same qualities you have demonstrated throughout your career.

You inspired me to become a better person. I genuinely want to be like you one day "when I grow up." There are no real superpowers per se, but your story is the closest I have heard to being a superhero in real life."

---

* All reflections were submitted by pre-medical and current medical students who participated in the original presentation of the ideas above.

"Thank you for sharing difficult stories about surgeries that went wrong and your thoughts and feelings in these situations. Your empathy and care for your patients and their loved ones is apparent."

"I was moved to tears by your account of your interaction with a patient's daughter after a devastating loss and found your emphasis on the human aspect of medicine incredibly touching. I felt a sense of relief and clarity because those kinds of experiences with the complexity and beauty of humanity are precisely what I perceived was lacking in my previous trajectory. For some, science just for the sake of science might be fulfilling enough based on the intellectual challenge, but to me, scientific research just feels meaningless and self-serving on its own. I feel solidified in my belief that medicine is the highest service and life's commitment to science. Although it has taken me a long time to feel worthy of it, I am more motivated than ever to become a compassionate and empathetic physician."

"Is this worth it?" And I'm sure you've faced this question many times throughout your career.

What I learned most from your talk was that sometimes, you have to be bold in going above and beyond. Perhaps not all surgeries are mind-blowing cases, or maybe your colleagues are telling you it's not necessary to respond to a patient's upset daughter—but I guess things do work out when you take the extra step."

"I truly enjoyed your talk. I don't believe I have ever had the opportunity to talk to a doctor who is as accomplished and compassionate as you.

It brought me to tears to hear you discuss your experience with the two patients you brought up in your case studies and hear just how vital each patient you have is to you, regardless of background or how small the issue may look to other doctors. You solidified why I want to go into medicine and become a surgeon."

"From the bottom of my heart, I am truly grateful for you. Your messages were insightful and empathetic, and your bravery is why I want to go into medicine. Thank you so much. I can't wait to get to touch not only patients' lives but also their family members' lives."

"Thank you for the invaluable and enriching information and personal experiences you've shared. Not only did I learn tremendously about the carotid endarterectomy procedure, but I also found it fascinating. I enjoyed seeing the emotional side of medicine, which is often taboo. Thank you for your authenticity and vulnerability in sharing such a poignant personal experience with us students. "

"I loved learning how William Silen, MD, taught you that a good surgeon builds a strong relationship with his/her patients and is also a good internist. Being disconnected was always one of my biggest reservations about surgery. Hearing you speak about the importance of a career as a physician was reinvigorating and reminded me of why I'm working as hard as I am to begin my career."

"This was a good reminder that, as a doctor, you never stop learning!

Everyone says, "The patient is human, and you must treat them as such," almost like it's a cliché. Your passion and drive for your patients were evident, and you gave such moving examples. It's also a very pertinent reminder that treating the patient usually isn't limited to the patient alone but affects their family and loved ones. And they need the same care and love that the actual patient requires because they, just like the doctor and the patient, are human too."

"You were heart-warming and reminded me how important compassion is to medicine. I find it easy to get separated from the idea of working with patients. Still, you reminded me of the importance of that human connection.

Many of my patients want someone to listen, address their fears/concerns, and make a compassionate connection. I am so glad to hear that there are physicians out there who give back to the community and help those who can so easily fall through the cracks. I hope to be a physician someday to give back to the community as you have with your patients and inspire young physicians."

"I can only hope to be as strong, humble, and compassionate as you one day."

About the Author

Richard A. Lynn, MD, FACS, RPVI, is a Phi Beta Kappa graduate of The Washington Square College of Arts and Sciences of New York University and the prestigious Cornell University Medical College. He completed residencies in surgery at the Beth Israel Hospital/Harvard Medical School and the Roosevelt Hospital/Columbia University College of Physicians and Surgeons. He practiced Vascular/Endovascular/General/Oncological Surgery in West Palm Beach, Florida, for 37 years.

Dr Lynn was artistic in his youth and attended The Arts Students League of New York. This later attracted him to the craft of surgery, as he understands surgery is an art.

Dr Lynn was recently honored by the American College of Surgeons as its Second Vice President. In 2017, Weil Cornell Medical School created the "Richard A. Lynn, MD '71 Scholarship," which is generously funded by grateful benefactors annually.

Dr Lynn lives in Palm Beach with his wife Margrit and their two dogs, Bella and Bessie. He is the proud father of three Orthodox Rabbi sons, twenty grandchildren, and five great-grandchildren. He is an avid reader and loves drumming.

Made in United States
Orlando, FL
02 August 2025

63484492R00062